Eternal Youth Secrets: How to Have Beautiful Hair, Glowing Skin at Any Age.

By VICKI TUONG VI, NGOC ANH, MINH TRANG

Healing H.A.P.P.Y. Bubbles Systems™

Modern Good Fortune, Prosperity, and Longevity:
"Live Hundreds of Years in a 30-year-old Body!"

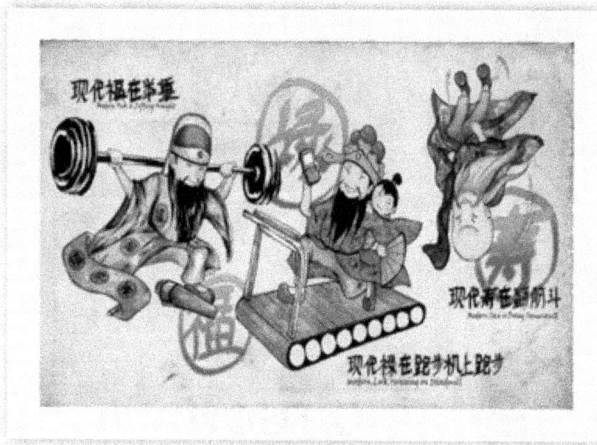

MAP OF CONSCIOUSNESS

God-view	Life-view	Level	Log	Emotion	Process
Self	Is	Enlightenment	700 1000	Ineffable	Pure Consciousness
All-Being	Perfect	Peace	↑ 600	Bliss	Illumination
One	Complete	Joy	↑ 540	Serenity	Transfiguration
Loving	Benign	Love	↑ 500	Reverence	Revelation
Wise	Meaningful	Reason	↑ 400	Understanding	Abstraction
Merciful	Harmonious	Acceptance	↑ 350	Forgiveness	Transcendence
Inspiring	Hopeful	Willingness	↑ 310	Optimism	Intention
Enabling	Satisfactory	Neutrality	↑ 250	Trust	Release
Permitting	Feasible	Courage	↓ 200	Affirmation	Empowerment
Indifferent	Demanding	Pride	↓ 175	Scorn	Inflation
Vengeful	Antagonistic	Anger	↓ 150	Hate	Aggression
Denying	Disappointing	Desire	↓ 125	Craving	Enslavement
Punitive	Frightening	Fear	↓ 100	Anxiety	Withdrawal
Disdainful	Tragic	Grief	↓ 75	Regret	Despondency
Condemning	Hopeless	Apathy	↓ 50	Despair	Abdication
Vindictive	Evil	Guilt	↓ 30	Blame	Destruction
Despising	Miserable	Shame	20	Humiliation	Elimination

Eternal Youth Secrets: How to Have Beautiful Hair and Glowing Skin at any Age

By
Vicki Tuong Vi, Ngoc Anh and Minh Trang

Graphics written and edited in USA and Vietnam

Disclaimer—Please Read!

The information in this book, workbook and videos are for your general knowledge and educational purposes only. This information has not been evaluated by the Food and Drug Administration. This book is not a substitute for medical advice or any treatments for specific medical conditions.

The materials and products on our websites are provided "as is" and without warranties of any kind, whether expressed or implied. These are not intended to diagnose, treat, cure, or prevent any disease. The authors shall not be liable for any special or consequential damages that result from the use of, misuse of, or the inability to use the materials on this book, workbook, DVD or the performance of the products[1].

The views, opinions, techniques, and products expressed in this workbook are those of the authors and do not necessarily reflect any official policy or position of any agencies or scientific or medical practices.

Examples and demonstrations performed within this workbook are only examples and illustrations. Techniques used within the book, workbook; videos only express the views and opinions of the authors and demonstrators. There is no scientific evidence or proof or research to prove that these examples and techniques are working for any individual.

Practice all techniques with caution. If you develop skin irritations or intense pain while using these products, stop using them immediately and consult your medical doctor.

---

[1] http://www.compwellness.org/notices.htm

Pregnant women, the elderly and children should not practice the acupressure method. Keep all referenced products out of the reach of children.

If you have any questions about your own health, skin, illnesses, diseases, or injuries, please seek advice from your personal medical professionals.

Table of Contents

Eternal Youth Secrets: How to Have Beautiful Hair, Glowing Skin at Any Age

Our body is an incredible organic machine. Biologically, spiritually, emotionally, and intellectually, it needs love, happiness, and to be nurtured with respect. It also needs nutrition, air, sunshine, water, and a balanced pH to function properly.

It needs about 14 vitamins and a host of 76 minerals and trace minerals [2], EFA, Amino Acids and thousands of enzymes (protein compound catalysts for metabolic and digestive processes). The 14 vitamins include the following: vitamin A, vitamin B-complex (8 types), vitamin C, vitamin D, vitamin E, and vitamin K2. The primary minerals include the following: calcium, chloride, copper, magnesium, phosphorus, potassium, sodium, and sulfur. Major trace minerals include the following: chromium, copper, fluoride, iodine, iron, manganese, molybdenum, selenium, and zinc.

Our body needs water to function. We are 70% plus water, so replenish water by drinking "clean water" daily. Water flushes toxins out of vital organs, carries nutrients to your cells, and provides a moist environment for ear, nose, and throat tissues. [3]

---

[2] http://www.mighty-90.com/the-90-essential-nutrients/
[3] http://en.wikipedia.org/wiki/Composition_of_the_human_body

Our body needs clean air. Pay attention to your breathing habits. Breathe deeply in, exhale out slowly. Make deep breathing your habit. Be happy, smile; feel the grace of living happily. Holding a pencil horizontally between your teeth is an exercise that can induce smiling and thus good feelings.

On the surface, skin is one of the most important aspects. It is the largest organ on the outside of your body, it protects everything inside. It is considered a detoxification organ and regulates body temperature. Other functions of the skin include sensation (transmits the surrounding conditions to the brain); immunity (helps the immune system); aids in expansion and movement; and the synthesis of vitamin D_3 on the skin to help with hormone balance (the endocrine system) of the body[4].

Our job is to give our skin proper nutrition and loving care so it can continue to function efficiently to allow us to stay younger and live longer in balance and harmony. The idea is not to take all the dietary supplements available or to eat the most expensive and most exotic foods, organic fruits, and vegetables.

The idea is to learn to know what your body needs by communicating with it. Getting to know your body is a skill acquired by muscle testing and by observation. Keeping a daily foods journal, and writing down thoughts and feelings will help you have a clear picture of what to provide for the needs of your emotional, mental, spiritual, and physical body.

---

[4] http://www.ivyroses.com/HumanBody/Skin/Functions-of-the-Skin.php

Your Body Demands You to Give What It Needs to Continue to Function

Step 1: Knowing the tools and the goals – Choose to be happy healthy.

Step 2: Understand nutrition and supplements. When your body does not have the nutrition it needs; it will take resources from itself for you to survive. In other words, it will eat itself to death! For example, in osteoporosis, mineral and calcium are taken away from the bones, making them hollow and breakable.

Step 3: Integration ☺ – Do daily – eat daily – happy daily – Know how to release stress and remember to love.

Step 4: Continue growth with fun and repeat the cycle of happy, healthy living.

The subject of this book and DVD is to care for your face and head (your hair, scalp, ears, etc.) and to learn how to keep them fresh, young, energetic, healthy, and make them even more beautiful every day. If the eyes are the windows to the soul, then the face is the reflection of your health. The methods in this book will allow you to create a routine caring for your face and head and allow them to *"be the ambassador for your being!"*

Choose to be healthy and beautiful inside out, and then take action. Incorporate the steps in your daily routine and see the magic happen!

We use *unique East and West techniques* (patent pending)— massaging, exercising, acupressure points and energy synchronizing — for the face and head. Face Acupressure is based on traditional Oriental acupressure points—it indeed has thousands of years of beauty secrets![5]

We recommend using only the purest lotions and creams— organic essential oils and natural herbs, vitamins for your skin and body. We believe it is better this way, as the human body is a biological system and would enjoy these healing natural resources. However, there may be some diverse effects — be sure to test them in small amounts first.

Finding the needs of your physical body is a skill that one must learn to master. After you learn the steps, fulfilling the needs to keep yourself in total health becomes a habit. It involves connecting with yourself, the unknown, and opening yourself up to invisible sources.

In our opinion, **Muscle Testing** or Applied Kinesiology (AK) is one of the best tools, if not the best tool, to use to find out what is good for each individual.

The step-by-step demonstration and instructions in this workbook and the DVD will amaze you. With simple tools such as your hands, you will discover that it is possible to have beautiful skin regardless of age. Using organic products for hair coloring, face creams, and cosmetics are unlikely to interfere with your body's processing the nutrition it needs for optimum health.

---

[5] http://en.wikipedia.org/wiki/Otzi_the_Iceman

This book: *Eternal Youth Secrets: How to Have Beautiful Hair and Glowing Skin At Any Age* is the first book in the series of *Healing H.A.P.P.Y. Bubbles* systems ™; which focuses on self-healing techniques in conjunction with Earth and Universal (Divinity) powers in synergy with human energies.

The techniques, programs, and processes are a combination of unique Energy Healing Systems called *Healing H.A.P.P.Y Bubbles* (*H*=Happy, *A*=Awesome, *P*=Phenomenal, *P*=Powerful, and *Y*=You) created for people to have a spiritual, safe, and private place for self-healing and self-care. They are praying systems without borders and limitations.

We also combine other modalities such as Sound Healing, Solfeggio Notes, Binaural Beats, Herbal Products and Vibrations, Essential Oils, Chakras Balancing, Quantum Harmonizing, EFT (Emotional Freedom Technique), Self-Generating Healing Protocols, Clearing Traumas, Nadis Massaging and much more.[6]

By learning **and applying energy healing**, you can have beauty inside and out. We are all vibrations. You may not be utilizing all of the forces available to you all the time. You may be missing out on many splendid mechanisms. Healing with energy can help you to achieve healthy and beautiful skin quickly and easily.

---

[6] https://en.wikipedia.org/wiki/Nadi_%28yoga%29

ONLY YOU CAN BREATHE FOR YOU, EAT FOR YOU OR GO TO THE BATHROOM FOR YOU → ONLY YOU CAN HEAL YOURSELF → YOU CAN ASK FOR HELP; THERE IS PLENTY OF THEM TO HEAL YOURSELF.

➤ Self-Healing is to understand your relationship with your SELF.
➤ Understand and Accept, Allow and Receive help.
➤ It is essential for good health, including skin health and total health.
➤ Beware of negative energies you allow into your life – Ask the Universe to transform, transmute, and transcend into beautiful energies, harming no one.

This system is for both men and women of all ages. Taking care of your hair, face, and mouth is what we all do every day. Take a few minutes in the morning before getting out of bed, and a few more minutes in the evening before sleeping, to breathe deeply, to relax, and to allow balance, beauty, and harmony into the SELF. Should be easy enough to do, right?

Learn how to deal with negative energies. Release them to Divinity to transform them and send back to the sender "10,000 blessings" instead of carrying the hurt, the betrayals, or the pains from them or from yourself.

We appreciate and thank you for your purchase. Our deepest desire when writing this book was to communicate with you that life is too long to live unhappily. Life is too long to live in suffering and pain.

This book is just the beginning of learning how to take good care of yourself. Your job is to learn to take good care of yourself; it is fundamental to good health. Once you learn to do it well, you can then take care of others with compassion, love, peace, and joy. And then we all can benefit.

Please use the book as a great gift of love for yourself. There is no greater gift than the gift of love and happiness. Use it as a gift of time for yourself. **There is no greater gift than the gift of beauty and time.**

In the last few decades, so many elderlies are suffering from the miseries of mental and physical illnesses. My friends and I had such parents, and we witnessed their sufferings, pains, and hopelessness in the human cycle of death.

We wonder if these are from the belief that a person is born, grows and dies with prewritten, unyielding faith. Does it come from our inner reptile brain striving for survival? The notion that people have to pay for their sins by suffering in old age, in loneliness and desperation is not a fun idea. The worst thing is that we have to come back, trying to learn, repeating the karma and the cycle of death again. And the circle of sufferings could restart again, in the "new" life. Sufferings can be in physical, emotional, mental, and spiritual forms.

December 12, 2012, the end of Maya calendar, has opened up a new dimension in awareness and spiritual growth for humanity. For us, it is the process and programming to connect and learn from Divinity (plug in the energies) to live life fully and beautifully today and every day [7]

We believe that aware, conscious, and spiritual adults have a different view of the limited human mechanism for survival. They believe that every human has choices. These spiritual beings can consciously create their own reality, and can choose to live life in abundance with dignity. When they decide to leave the physical body, they can go at their own chosen time with ease and grace, no fuss, no muss, no burden, and with celebration and happiness.

It is true, we also believe, in the end, that we are all in One. And everything is going to be okay. However, everyone has their choice of how to grow, when and where and in what circumstances. Some choose agonies, struggling through life until death to become oneness again.

In our opinion, the first reason for wanting miseries is the non-awareness of other alternatives. Of course, we can't choose for others, but we certainly can choose for ourselves. We can choose happy choices. We can decide to live and die with dignity and honor without suffering and without being a heavy load to society and our loved ones.

The second reason for a painful life is the disconnection with our spiritual universe and not asking for help. Many of us don't know how to ask, allow, accept, and receive assistance that is the most beneficial for the physical body.

The third reason is the inability to utilize the three energies of Divinity, Earth, and Human power to create your reality of desires and destiny.

---

[7] http://www.openhandweb.org/a_new_earth_is_born

For many years, we struggled with this book and the accompanying DVD, to describe how to share and spread the knowledge and techniques of natural healing to ease the pains and heal the hurt. We did not know how to share these secrets with you, with the world. We asked for help to find the ways...

Then we found them! **Amazing,** ask and you shall receive. When one opens up to the possibilities, there are wonders in front of one's eyes! These groups are always there; we don't know why we did not see them before. LOL.

We deeply thank Tammy, Mike, Barry, and Roger for sharing the world of caring and support. And for giving us encouragement and HOPE with fun to continue the sharing journey!

You see, **there are over 40+ skin disorders,** ranging from annoying little warts to embarrassing rosacea to devastating lupus and basal cancer.

Also, autism, diabetes, heart disease, cancer, Alzheimer, to name just a few, are disastrous to our happiness.

The fact is all of these lifelong disabilities could be prevented and in some cases could be cured totally. We, indeed, can have total health and happiness.

Good health and well-being give the ability to be independent, the capacity to have an impact on oneself and the world, and the skill to handle unlimited power with the responsibility to do good.

Think of the people you can help by opening up to learning natural healing combined with modern technologies:

➤ You can take superb care of yourself.

- ➤ You can help your children and the children of the world to better health.
- ➤ You can contribute to lessening the pain and hurt of ailing elderly, both yours and others.
- ➤ You can make the world a little bit brighter or a lot!

With that, we would like to invite you inventors, business owners, holistic professional, healers, entrepreneurs, teachers, trainers, consultants, coaches, students, moms, dads, speakers present and future authors, sponsors, affiliates, partners, people from all walks of life, to join the Divine Healing H.A.P.P.Y. Bubbles programs.

The goal is to explore the mystical, healthy choices for yourself and to live your life the beautiful way you desire.

And then spread the awareness to help others, to ease the pain and hurt of the sick and helpless.

Also to help the children, the future of human race, to know how to choose for themselves and to continue the legacy of dignity, truth, beauty, and grace.

And, when you are ready, to leave your physical body and depart with joy and peace at your personal chosen time and place.

Who Is this Book for?

The books and programs are for professional women and men from 30 to 50 years old, in 3 groups:

Making Conscious Choices of Love, Loving, and Being Loved

Love and respect yourself.
Love is the foundation of life, of all things. Love, being loved, and loving is essential for good health, good fortune, for everything in life.

---

1. Corporate professional men and women.

This group has the most responsibilities and the busiest schedules. If you are in this group, you are in the prime of your life. Your education is completed, and now you are working full-time in the workforce building a career. Some of your responsibilities might include the following:

- Knowing how to care for yourself so you can continue to be healthy to work and care for your world.
- Needing to have a good, professional appearance.
- You might have young children or elderly parents to care for.
- You might have to manage team members.
- ⇨ **Love with Respect is the focus here. Love is mandatory for Life; it could help you and your loved ones to have peace and joy of living!**

2. Actors, Actress, Hollywood celebrities

- You might have a need to present yourself in the most favorable way.
- You travel and have a busy demanding schedule, yet need to be calm, pleasant, and joyful.
- Your job is most stressful and unstable. You need to find your core to be in balance.
⇨ **Beauty with Integrity is the focus here. It could help you to have fun and enjoy the majesty of your being more every day.**

3. Public officials in organizations or government

- You are in the public eye and need to have a good, presentable appearance.
- You are busy, and demands are constant for you to deliver results at a high-performing level.
- You have a need for clarity, balance, and wisdom to make important decisions affecting many people and the world.
⇨ **Success with Honor and Happiness with Dignity is the focus here; it could enhance the fulfillment and satisfaction of your destiny.**

Baby Boomers Group: Perhaps this group needs Healing HAPPY Bubbles system the most! They might not have resources for better health. They might not have the decision power to do anything for themselves. However, it is never too late for positive changes, for taking actions to improve one's health!

We hope you can help!

Why Is It Important to be Aware of the Right Choice?

You are a member of these powerful groups that can make decisions and take actions that affect many people around you and in your life, including yourself.

The whole process comes down to a fundamental choice and awareness:

Do you choose to be healthy and happy to live your life, or do you choose to stay in a stressful, hurry-up-and-wait situation all the time?

The other side of choice is the power to *allow, accept, and receive* help from the Divine Teams and Earth rather than accept the values of the Suffering Gangs, such as illnesses, aches and pains, injuries, and negative emotions.

Awareness of human duality: It is said that human beings created duality to experience dark and light, right and wrong, suffering and enlightenment.

The physical body is an illusion and a field of frozen thoughts and matter, and it can be changed by healing the aura, mental, emotional, and spiritual bodies.

Sometimes, this healing is referred to as a *miracle*. Sometimes, it comes as a process.

Your physical body is one of the many bodies you have. There are multiple formations, multiple levels of energies, and much more that are invisible inside and outside and all around you. There are things that human beings can't do; we need help and intervention from the Divinity. We need Love from Earth.

You can combine what you are doing now with the techniques and processes in the book, workbook and DVD. The wonderful part is you can, in a few minutes, massage and exercise your face, your hands anytime and anywhere. ☺

These are simple and effective things that can add years of beauty and happiness to your life! Furthermore, you can add years of health to the lives of people you care about and love. To us, this is the biggest reward of being beautiful and healthy!

Series of weekly webinars:

The Eternal Youth Methods
Money Goodness with The Magic Scanner
Is available at

www.FunHappyStore.com

Learn how to transform energies into beneficial sources for your Health, Beauty and Wellness; including Creating Blessed Water, Clearing Traumas, Manifesting Wealth and much more!

Book Structure and Core Thoughts

❖ **The Book is written in an outcome-based format and is action driven. It includes:**

Chapter Summaries to clarify ideas and to induce actions.

Box Fun Facts and Comments of interesting thoughts, which promote simplicity and fun.

Brain thoughts in colors: [8] Multicolor, funny pictures, different fonts, to stimulate subconscious and unconscious curiosity and to help retain ability.

❖ **Core thought: We are all in One, but we are not the same.**

Each of us is a whole universe of consciousness unto itself. Each human is unique with our own physical self, talents, thoughts, mind, emotions, expressions, and consciousness.

The ability to synergy [9] with outside energies to your own depends on your awareness and choices. So, for this reason, the outcome of your health and happiness rely upon the decisions you make.

---

[8] http://bit.ly/1UKadMK

[9] https://www.google.com/search?q=synergy+with+other+or+to&ie=utf-8&oe=utf-8

❖ **Core thought:** **Have fun with responsibility: everything is okay, no matter what.**

> Learn **to make the Right Choice,** then help spread awareness and awakening to a higher dimension of living and dying.

> **Remember the Love**: Self-love, Love and to be Loved. Take care of yourself first, and then learn to take care of others and respect their choice, their privacy, and their boundaries.

> By praying without borders and asking Divinity to send them Love for No Reason, we can ease the pain and suffering of others instead of taking on their hurts and pains.

> In the same core thought, the Human Race is beautiful and eternal. It is here to continue to grow and expand, and it always has the support of the whole universe.

> **Expect healings, blessings and miracles**. Everything is okay. Everything will work out okay, so go ahead, have fun living angel vibrations in human form!

Okay, enough said; thank you for listening. Let the journey begin!

Chapter 1 — The Anatomy of Your Skin

Human skin is a part of the integumentary system. It is a live, biological machine. It covers the whole enchilada—the inside and outside of your body, all visible and invisible parts. **The real boss of your skin is your brain.**

Imagine your skin is the *outside* of your house. Outside, it has a roof and four walls with electrical connections, windows, maybe a balcony that is constantly exposed to the elements. The *inside* of your house has a foundation, an upstairs, downstairs, different rooms, furniture, stove, washing machine, refrigerators, etc.

You will need to keep up your house, outside and inside, so it is safe to live in. You need to respond to its needs by paying attention and taking proper actions.

The skin is alive; just like you are. It houses your physical body, aura, psychic body, intellectual body, mental body, emotional body, and spiritual body.

Skin needs to grow new cells and shed the old cells, which allows it to replace its surface every 27 days. Every hour, your skin sheds 600,000 particles. The dust under your sofa is your dead skin cells. However, you still must dust and clean your house!

The normal temperature of the skin is about 32 to 36 C or 90-96 F.

If the skin loses its ability to regenerate cells, it will become fragile and open to disorders.

Normal skin temperature is about 32 to 36 C or 90-96 F.

Every day, an adult body produces 300 billion new cells. It is, however, just a fraction of your 10 trillion total cells.

The skin has the ability to stretch and return to normal afterward, very elastic. Silica, a trace mineral, strengthens connective tissues and helps skin health.

Some research suggests the oil in your dead skin cells absorbs the toxins in the ozone and therefore improves the air.

For example, when the foundation of your house is faulty, or the walls break down, or the roof leaks, you must repair it.

In choosing a repairer to fix your house, you want to take into consideration the quality of his work, trustworthiness, reputation, and price point. After you repair your house, you need to maintain it.

The equivalent to selling your house to move to a new place is when you decide to die—leaving the present physical form to a different dimension of existence.

Your body is a whole universe itself, with trillions of cells in several organs. It has multiple functions and unlimited expansion. To care for it with love and respect is to honor your life; it will do the same for you.

You must nurture your skin in a similar way as taking care of your house. Choose herbals, quality, and natural products, including foods, water, and nutritional supplements from trustworthy, reputable companies with proven records to care for your skin.

If you have skin issues, take care of the problem, bring it to a healthy level, and then continue to maintain it.

The job of taking care of your skin does not have to be hard. It can be a joy, a beautiful place to live in and to laugh with joy and happiness.

Color and properties of the skin change with health and the age of a person. Winkles, marks, and liver spots come with aging and sun exposure.

Skin disorders from minor to severe conditions pose a danger to health and are the results of many factors: exposure to chemicals and harmful sun rays, nutritional deficiencies, and energy deprivation.

Knowing how to take care of your skin is not just about taking care of its surface on the outside; **it is about understanding and having an intimate relationship with your *whole being*** and connecting with the eternal Universe.

It is about knowing and choosing your choices consciously. It is a mystical and mysterious journey of living and loving. And it is a delightful, joyous thing to do!

Under the Skin: Muscles, Bones, & Brain, & Tons of other stuff.

Muscles: Human has more than 600 muscles with three different types: smooth, cardiac or heart, and skeletal muscles.

You have no conscious control of **smooth muscles or involuntary muscles**. They are inside your stomach, bladder, and even in the eyelids that keep the eyes focused.

Heart muscles are in the heart and they work automatically for you; however, they are influenced by other systems in order to function normally.

Skeletal muscles are the muscles directly under the skin. They connect with the bones to allow the body to move around.

Face muscles: there are 43 muscles in the face, controlled by facial nerves—they help to show emotions on the face and enable you to talk and swallow.

It takes 17 muscles to smile and 62 muscles to frown. Also, smiles create melatonin, the feel-good chemical in your body, so smile more often.

Muscles are fibrous tissues, and they use amino acids from protein to function and the amino acids need to be refilled to keep muscles in healthy condition

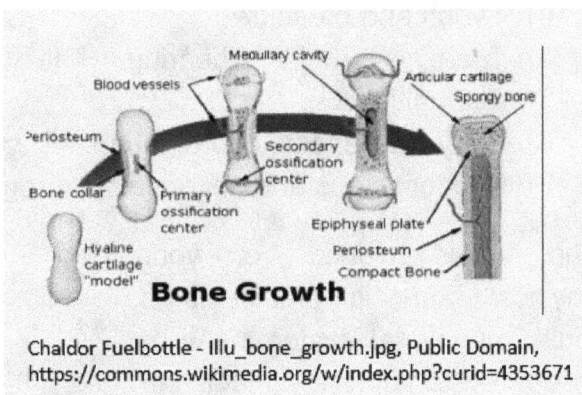

Bone Growth

Chaldor Fuelbottle - Illu_bone_growth.jpg, Public Domain, https://commons.wikimedia.org/w/index.php?curid=4353671

Bones are the frame of the body. Without bones, the body is just a pile of soft tissues, immobile and stuck in one place; unable to function in balance.

Babies are born with about 270 bones, and these bones become 206 bones in adults. Bones are made of collagen cells; they store minerals and vitamins. The marrow inside the bones has important functions in red blood cell regeneration.

The spine is the main bone connecting the skull and the arms and legs. When the spine joints are out of place, it will affect your overall health and mobility.

An important factor in caring for skin: understanding and working with the Mind and the BRAIN consciously!

The physical brain has many parts and many functions, some of them are:

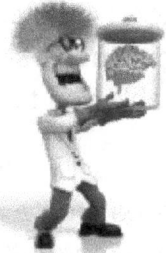

1) Concentration, planning, organization, problem solving.
2) Motor control, balance control.
3) Speech, vision, language, understanding, knowing.
4) Touch and pressure.
5) Taste, smell, hearing, facial recognition.
6) Body awareness, coordination.
7) Subconscious and unconscious programming.

The whole wonder of your physical body is that it is a multidimensional system. All of these systems are under an invisible command center: **The Brain!** The brain is a vessel; the mind is part of your Being. Connect the brain, mind, body, and spirit to the heart to harmonize your life.

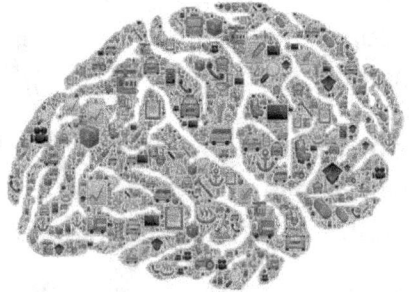

Pixabay.com free image brain 954823_640

The brain is like an operating system of a computer. It runs as it is programmed. To let this operating system run by itself is to give the **robot** total control of your life, to make it the **BOSS** without your conscience!

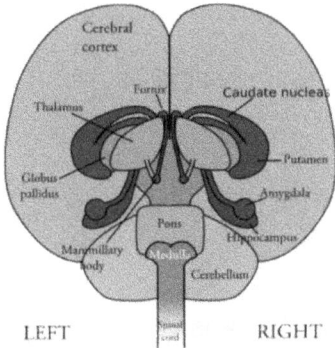

LEFT   RIGHT

Pixabay.com free image brain 40356_640

This boss can be a tyrant with constant demands and pressures. This boss can be laden with unresolved conflicts and unresolved dreams and desires. This tyrant's job is to hurt you, harm you, and even kill you.

On the other hand, **you can choose to be the boss of your life.** You have the power to choose and direct this gray matter to work with you! Then, this boss can be a loving, supporting partner of your life and health. It is not a boss. Instead, it is a **co-creator,** full with wisdom and divine intelligence; it is a part of your oneness. In other words, the brain is part of you.

In accepting the responsibility to be the co-creator for your life; embrace the help of Earth, Angels, Divinity, and honorable Humans to broaden your consciousness and freedom. Be a co-creator, selecting to learn the skills needed to be a valuable team player for your life, reality and Being!

Heal the Brain First

"A lot of us don't understand the importance of Brain Mind Body Spirit Integration!"

➤ **Physical brain health:** this physical brain needs: oxygen, protein, fat (ketones), sugar (glucose), vitamins, minerals and trace minerals. The physical brain is part of the mind. It's like the hardware of computer; running as programmed.
But it is much more complex in humans. Without the automated brain, we can't function "normally!"

➤ **Emotional brain:** needs safety, expansion understanding and love,

➤ **Etheric brain or mind needs:** goodness, purposes, beauty, continuation, connection. The mind is everywhere and in every cell. It makes choices and decisions affecting the individual. It is part of the soul. It is consciousness, perception, judgement and memory.

➤ **Spiritual brain or Truer SELF needs:** Co-creation, clarity, synergy Earth, Divinity, Human energy, truth, vision, happiness, teamwork for the Highest Good of All.

Chapter 1: The Anatomy of Your Skin — Summary Box

1. Choose to have beautiful, healthy skin. Proactively care for your skin as it is the frontier of your health.

2. Skin protects everything in our bodies: muscles, tissues, blood vessels, nerves, bones, and organs from exposure to hash environmental elements including trauma, radiation, toxins, and bacteria.

3. Hair and nails are part of the skin systems. They share a similar chemical makeup but serve different functions as part of your physical body.

4. Taking good care of your skin means knowing the difference between YOU and your BRAIN, including loving yourself and your total (7) bodies of your Being, including the physical environment, foods, air, water, dietary supplements, and related items.

5. Carefully choose natural herbs and quality dietary supplements from reputable, trustworthy companies. Synthetic and chemical-filled products will accumulate toxins inside your body and could do more harm than good.

6. Integration: be the best you can be. Understand your skin's language. Symptoms and physical pain are the ways your skin communicates with you, telling you it needs nutrition. Cleanse it to be back in balance.

7. Grow and have fun: Continue to help your skin become healthy and more beautiful every day and grow your awareness of and awakening to learning and using Energy Healing as part of your life.

Chapter 2 — Understanding Your Skin Inside Out

Skin Layers

Skin is the large, outer organ of the *integumentary system* that includes the skin, nails, and hair. It is a multifunctional organ. It has different thicknesses depending on its location and the functions of the organs underneath it.

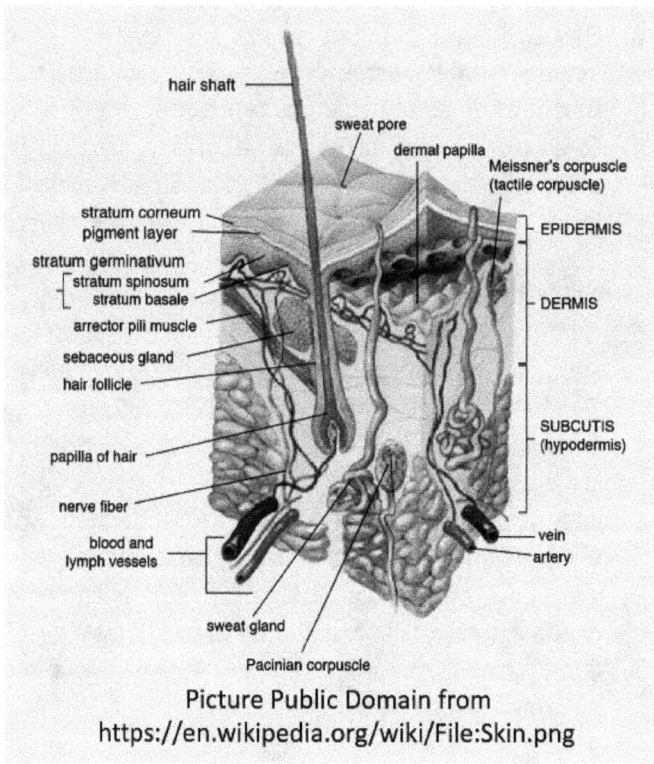

hair shaft

sweat pore

dermal papilla

Meissner's corpuscle (tactile corpuscle)

stratum corneum
pigment layer

EPIDERMIS

stratum germinativum
stratum spinosum
stratum basale

DERMIS

arrector pili muscle

sebaceous gland

hair follicle

SUBCUTIS (hypodermis)

papilla of hair

nerve fiber

blood and lymph vessels

vein

artery

sweat gland

Pacinian corpuscle

Picture Public Domain from
https://en.wikipedia.org/wiki/File:Skin.png

There are three main layers of skin; inside each layer, there are additional strata (layers) the epidermis, the dermis, and the hypodermis.

1). The outermost layer of the skin is **the epidermis**. It functions as a protective shield. It is waterproof, but when immersed in water for a long time, it can become wrinkled and easily damaged. It has many functions: protect, regulate temperature; a sensor to the brain; absorption, secretion, elimination; and vitamin synthesis.

Inside the epidermis, there are four layers:

1) **Cornified (stratum corneum)** has 20 to 30 cell layers, is waterproof, and protects against chemical and physical assaults.
2) **Stratum lucidum is the clear/translucent layer** found only on the palms of hands and soles of the feet. It is thick skin because it has 5 epidermis layers instead of 4.

On the average, your skin covers 21 square feet, (about 2 square meters), carrying 11 miles of blood vessels. Adult skin weighs around eight lbs. or over 3.5 kilograms.

Skin is a continuous organ outside the body Inside the skin; there are mucous membranes, lining other organs. Mucus membranes are large, about 400 square meters and are very vulnerable. They include the lining of the mouth, nose, anus, urethra, and vagina.

Skin is individual to each person, and each person's skin has its pigment, skin tone, color (melanin), and growth rate. When we are sick or have a nutritional deficiency, the skin will vividly reflect this condition.

The thinnest epidermis is on the eyelid, .05 mm. The thickest skin is on the palms of the hands and the soles of our feet, at 1.5.mm.

3) **Granular layer (stratum granulosum) and the spinous layer (stratum spinosum).** They have keratin, a fibrous protein, which gives the skin strength and flexibility and is waterproof. Keratin makes up most of the hair and keeps hair from becoming dry and damaged. **Spinous layer (stratum spinosum).** It has keratin, a fibrous protein, which gives the skin strength and flexibility and is waterproof. Keratin makes up most of the hair and keeps it from becoming dry and damaged.

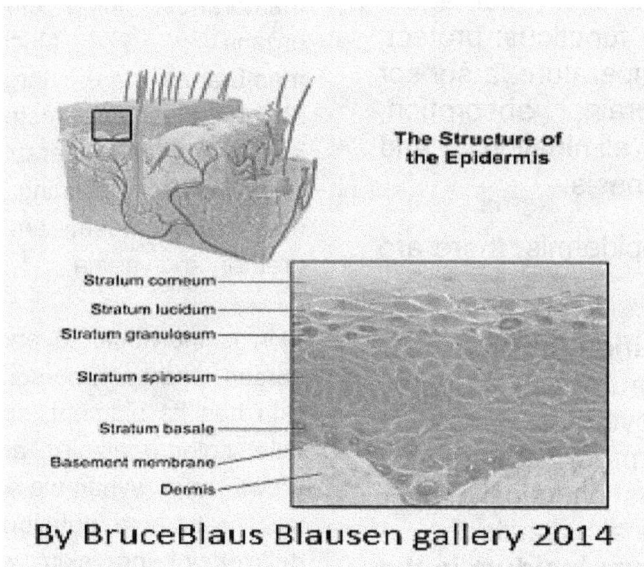

The Structure of
the Epidermis

Stratum corneum
Stratum lucidum
Stratum granulosum
Stratum spinosum
Stratum basale
Basement membrane
Dermis

By BruceBlaus Blausen gallery 2014

4) **Basal/germinal layer (stratum basale/germinativum),** the deepest layer of the 4 layers, contains basal cells. Basal cells produce new skin cells as the old ones die. This is the deepest layer of the epidermis. UV light causes skin damage to this layer that can lead to basal cell carcinoma. This skin cancer is easily treated in its early stage but it is not to be ignored.[10]

---

[10] https://en.wikipedia.org/wiki/Epidermis

The dermis thickness on the eyelid is 0.3mm and 3.0mm on the back.

When skin lacks amino fatty acids, it becomes dry and cracks easily, causing permanent scars. Scars can be removed or minimized in many ways. For example: massaging, stretching, deep tissue massaging, using cream to dissolve the dead tissues, and laser surgery.

Subcutaneous fat is not necessarily as harmful as visceral fat is. *Visceral fat,* or abdominal fat, accumulates around your organs. It interferes with nutrients' absorption. Visceral fat has been linked to diabetes and heart disease. It can be measured using the Bio-Tracker scale from Nature's Sunshine.

2). The dermis: second layer of the skin. It functions to provide structure and support. It is the cushion, protecting the body from stress and strain.

It is beneath the epidermis and has two layers: the **papillary dermis,** which has loose collagen fibers; and the **reticular dermis,** the fatty layer found in connective tissue, nerve endings, oil glands, hair follicles, sweat glands, receptors, nails, and blood circulation.[11]

The dermis has three types of cells: fibroblasts (extracellular matrix and collagen) that are critical in healing wounds; macrophages (white blood cells that fight against toxins); and adipocytes (energy tissue stored as fat).

---

[11] https://en.wikipedia.org/wiki/Dermis

3) **The hypodermis** or subcutaneous is the third tier. It functions as insulation to slow down heat loss, acts to pad the skin against shock and friction, and anchors the skin to the inside of the body.

The hypodermis is the thickest layer of the skin. It stores the skin's energy reserves of collagen and fibrous fiber. Aging causes thinning of the hypodermis layer, leading to drooping skin, the forming of skin folds, wrinkles, and sagging of the face. The fat-storing cells, *adipocytes*, are grouped together by connection tissues. This fat is most noticeable on the shoulders and stomachs of men and the buttocks, thighs, and hips of women.[12]

This unhealthy visceral fat can be measured with the Bio-Tracker of IN.FORM program with Nature's Sunshine.

I love this scientific approach, and I am currently an IN.FORM certified coach.

The cool thing about the program is it goes to the root cause of the good health problem – the gut health or microbiome which affects everything in the human body, as demonstrated in this picture:

---

[12] http://dynamicnaturesite.blogspot.com/2012/12/hypodermis-layer-function.html

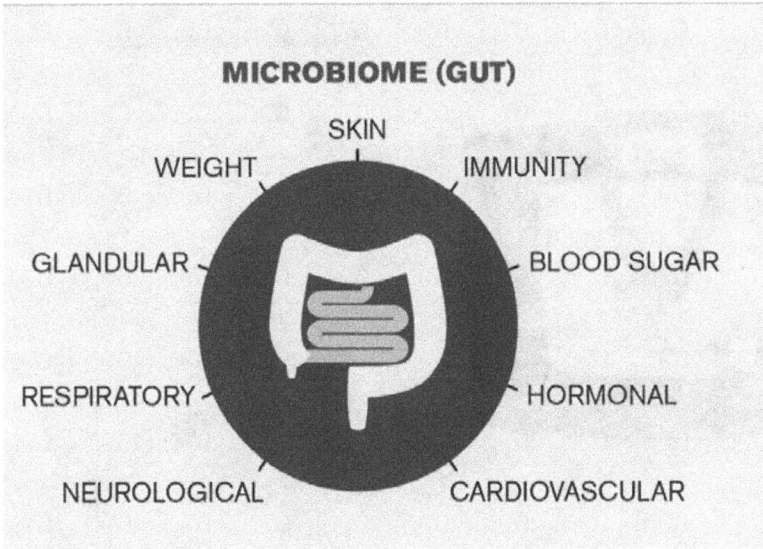

MICROBIOME (GUT)

SKIN

WEIGHT — IMMUNITY

GLANDULAR — BLOOD SUGAR

RESPIRATORY — HORMONAL

NEUROLOGICAL — CARDIOVASCULAR

The IN.FORM Bio-Tracker illustrated below is a device that measures metabolic age, associated with the effectiveness of your metabolism. It should be similar to your biological age or lower.

Vicki's biological age is 68; her metabolic age was 36 at the time this book was written! [13]

The IN.FORM program is a unique health maintenance course, to track important markers to be fit, healthier and happier for life!

---

[13] IN.FORM - Nature's Sunshine Products. (n.d.). Retrieved from https://www.naturessunshine.com/us/members/c1/inform-weight-management1/why-info

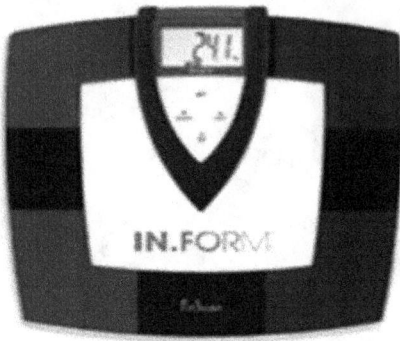

MEASUREMENTS
Weight
Body Fat %
Body Water %
Muscle Mass
DCI (Daily Caloric Intake)
Metabolic Age
Bone Mass
Visceral Fat
Chest
Waist
Hips
Thigh
Bicep
Neck

For more information about the program, please contact: Vicki Tuong Vi Eaton – IN.FORM Coach – FunHappyStore.com

The Inner Skin – Mucus membranes
Mucus membranes are the slippery secretions that line and protect various organs. Their functions are to fight pathogens and prevent the tissues in the body from drying up. When mucus membranes dry up, the cells stick together, and the organs can't function or absorb nutrition, possibly causing many diseases.

They are also found between eyes and the ears. The human body produces about a half of a liter of mucus every day. [14]

---

[14] https://www.naturessunshine.com/content/us/misc/webinar/EdWk-Feb16-Skinny-on-Snot.pdf

Skin Is a Sophisticated Sensory Organ

The Senses. The head and the face are the most exposed parts of the body. The brain is the command center of all our beings and our senses, both conscious and unconscious. There are twelve system senses; 7 known and 5 unknowns. The seven known senses are: 1. touch (tactile or somatosensory system), 2. movement (proprioception system), 3. smell (olfactory system), 4. taste (gustatory system), 5. sight (visual system), 6. hearing (auditory system) and 7. balance (vestibular system).

These senses are highly specific yet interdependent and affect each other in the sensory integration system, thereby making it possible for us to use our body efficiently and automatically.

Also, there are several different dimensions to the sensory integration system.

1) **The tactile system (touch)** has two distinct levels: discrimination determines where the touch is and what is touching the body. The second tier is sometimes called the "fight or flight" response (the reaction to stress: run away or stay and fight back). These two levels must work in harmony for the interpretation of information and survival.

The proprioceptive (movement) system: These are receptors that respond to muscle contractions and the stretching of joints and tendons. This system is involved in providing awareness to the body and to keep track of your position and your balance from the acceleration and flexibility of external forces. It is a feedback mechanism for motor control and posture. Along with the vestibular system in the inner ear, it helps keep the body oriented and balanced.[15]

The brain automatically utilizes this constant influx of sensory information. It sends out mental adjustments, along with beliefs embedded in the subconscious, to respond. Sometimes, this is referred to as the sixth sense, developed by the nervous system as an automatic and "permanent" mechanism.

2) **Smell (olfactory system):** through the specialized sensory cells in the nasal system. Human smell is much less sensitive than that of animals. However, it is still very amazing, especially when the smell is connected with emotions and traumas. Then it becomes a part of the person's personality.

The smell sense also relates to breathing in and out by mouth and nose. Allergies are reactions in the nasal and immune systems that respond to air pollutants and harmful chemicals.

3) **Taste (gustatory system):** is composed of taste buds on the tongue, roof, and side of the mouth and throat. There are about 2000 to 5000 taste buds with seven tastes: sour, bitter, sweet, salty, pungent (spicy), astringent and umami (savory taste). Foods and culture has an enormous influence on taste, and closely associated with the sense of smell and sight.

---

[15]   http://cherringtonsawers.com/tactile-vestibular-and-proprioceptive-senses.html

4) **Sight (visual system)** is the dominant human sense. In the vestibular system, sight is a major component. Twenty percent of neurons in the visual system react to the balance or vestibular stimulation. (e.g., when spinning, head shaking, or rocking).

> Vision is the process of measuring and deriving the meaning of seeing images. Its primary purpose is to come up with an appropriate response to the immediate or future situation.

> Researchers estimate eighty or more percent of perceptions, learning, cognition, and activities and pleasures are by vision.

> Newborn babies see upside down until the brain learns to process it right side up.

5) **Hearing (the auditory system):** an important sense in translations and communication to keep us upright.

> There are two sets of end organs in the inner ear, or labyrinth: the semicircular canals, which respond to rotational movements and the otoliths. Anything that disrupts the sense of auditory information could affect the vestibular function. For example, ear diseases could cause balancing issues.

Sound waves move into the ear canal until they reach the eardrums. They then pass into the inner ear with many tiny ear hairs, which pass on the sounds to the brain. The brain interprets the sounds and sends the information back to you. Music affects people deeply on many levels can cause either extreme discomfort or pleasure.

6) **Balance (Vestibular System)** Balance is the sense of orientation (up, down, left, right, horizontal, vertical, etc.) and the gravity relationship with the earth and other objects in space. It tells the body whether it is moving, how fast, and in what direction (forward, backward, etc.)

   It controls head position and movements, coordination, eye movement, and your attention span, including some language developments.

Other components provide sensory information to the vestibular system: **hands, fingers, and pressure on the soles of the feet provide information about the texture of the ground.**

Dysfunctions in the vestibular system can cause anxiety, nausea, a need for self-stimulation, abnormalities in muscle tone, and academic problems.[16]

Notes: Belly breathing, deep breathing, meditations, and sounds are ways of relaxing muscles and movements that release stress (centering the Self). Smiling, rolling the eyes, and stretching the mouth also efficiently release the tension on the face.

---

[16] http://www.spdaustralia.com.au/the-vestibular-system/

Chapter 2: Understanding Your Skin Inside Out— Summary Box

1. The seven known senses—touch, (proprioceptive) movement, smell, taste, sight, hearing, and (vestibular) balance—are all connected to the brain, all inner organs, and the skin.

2. Education, social settings, cultures, personal references and different levels of consciousness have a significant impact on human senses. Choices of foods, clothing, music, spouse, and even business partners reflect these influences.

3. There are three main layers of skin:
    a. Epidermis (has four sublayers); its functions include: temperature regulation, absorption, protection, secretion, elimination, sensation, and vitamin D3 synthesis.
    b. Dermis (has two sublayers); it gives the skin its elasticity, strength, flexibility, and support. It has nerve endings, hair roots, oil glands, receptors, and nail and blood vessels.
    c. Hypodermis, the thickest layer of the skin, stores fat that can be converted to energy.
    d. Mucous membranes line the inside skin and help protect and fight against infection and connects various organs.

4. The skin has several functions and needs. Give it nutrients and good care so it can continue to perform for you at an optimal level.

5. *IN.FORM Nature's Sunshine health program: is a unique and effective course to understand the relationship of physical body and skin and health* ☺

Chapter 3—Factors Affecting Skin Health

External Environment

The face and head are the most exposed to the sun. The neck, arms, and hands are also regularly exposed to the environment.

The *environment* includes everything around you: air pollutants, contaminated water, toxins in cleaning products, smoke, noise, sun exposure, harsh weather, improper skin care, and toxins in skin care products. We are exposed to harmful chemicals much more today than 20 or even 10 years ago.

Household toxic chemicals: These toxins could severely affect health, especially in young children, homemakers, and the elderly who are home all day.

There are about 40+ skin disorders including the following: acne, cold sores, rashes, diaper rash, warts, psoriasis, hives, vitiligo, canker sores, eczema, nail fungus, fungal infections, flaky scalps, herpes, necrotizing fasciitis, ingrown nails, cutaneous candidiasis, impetigo, measles, rosacea, lupus, and skin cancer.

We recommended holistic processes to cure skin disorders:
1) Decide to be healthy.
2) Ask the question: "What is the root cause, feedback, and message?"
3) Eliminate the culprit (use all the tools: modern, herbal, clearing traumas, praying selectively).
4) Bring balance and harmony.
5) Let go of the past.
6) Vision bright future.
7) Maintain healthy status

> The toxins are continuously exposed to them.[17] *Take precautions: wear gloves when washing dishes, and open windows to air out cleaner's fumes.*

> **Learn to read UPC codes:** Avoid chemicals and artificial ingredients. **GMO** is a process that denotes that food products have been genetically modified and is highly controversial [18]

UPC code 5 digit on produce: Number 9 prefix indicates the produce is organically grown – For example: #94011 is organic yellow banana. [19]

UPC code on products is 12 digits: Number 00-09 is from USA and Canada. The number: 690-692 is from China. From France: 30-37. Number 40-44 is from Germany. 471 from Taiwan. 50 is UK. 49 is Japan. [20]

A sample of Nature's Harvest vegetable protein drink UPC code is below.

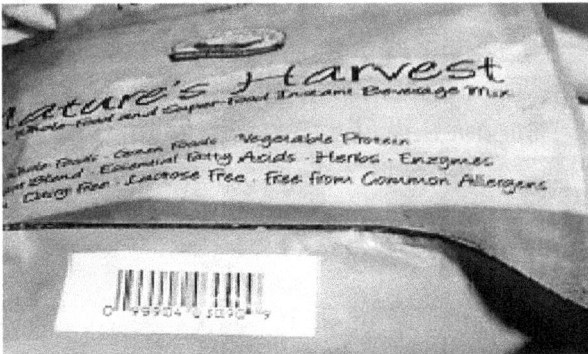

---

[17] http://www.shareguide.com/hazard.html
[18] http://www.wholefoodsmarket.com/gmo-quick-facts-what-why-where
[19] http://ww2.kqed.org/bayareabites/2012/11/20/food-labeling-how-to-identify-conventional-organic-and-gmo-produce/
[20] https://www.nationwidebarcode.com/barcodes-where-products-come-from/

➢ **Read the product label for ingredients, process and origin**: Some of the deceiving words to avoid in ingredients are: High Fructose Corn Syrup, Partially Hydrogenated Oils, Sodium Nitrate, Aspartame, Sucralose, MSG (Monosodium Glutamate), Artificial Flavors, Artificial Coloring, Soy Lecithin.[21]

Radiation that was used on imported products could destroy their natural nutrition. Knowing where products are from should also be taken into consideration for quality and nutritional values.

➢ **Harmful sunlight** is probably the most dangerous condition for skin. It can cause permanent damage such as freckles, age spots, rough skin, and skin cancer.

"Photo-aging" is the aging of the hands, face, ears, and neck caused by UVA and UVB rays.

UVA—Ultraviolet rays type A penetrate deep into the skin and destroy the collagen, elastin, and the fiber matrix, which support the skin. Constant exposure to UVA rays causes the dermis to be thinner, leads to drooping skin, and the formation of deep folds in the skin called wrinkles. Also, it affects the growth of the cells and could lead to severe skin disorders like lupus and skin cancer.

UVB – Ultraviolet rays type B cause changes to the skin pigments as you get tan and probably sunburn, too. Sunburn makes the dermis thinner, with discomfort and itching, and could cause breaks in the skin with infections.

---

[21] www,informnsp.com

Always use organic sunscreen to help protect the skin. Apply it daily. Do not use sunscreen with harmful chemicals.

There is some controversy about using creams that contain the new technologies of nanoparticles (microscopic particles) and their effect on the skin. Nanoparticles absorb quickly into the skin and disappear, and could cause harmful reactions inside the body.

Non-nanoparticles in creams stay on the skin and need to be massaged in the skin or evened out on the skin surface to protect it. Eventually, it is washed off without any systemic effect.

> **Lifestyles and habits (drinking, smoking, taking in other's pains and sufferings)**

Drinking and substance abuse that causes breakdowns in your liver and spleen functions will also affect your skin.

Smoking with nicotine intake speeds up the breakdown of skin cells and causes breathing and lung damage. It is common knowledge that smokers look older and have more wrinkles than nonsmokers.

Loud, unpleasant noises cause vibrations deep at the cellular level. They can damage your hearing, cause sleep deprivation, and stress.

Humans have many needs. One of them is the need to belong. Many times, when we need to belong to a group, an organization, we want to fit in and share the emotions. A lot of times, movies, books and news can affect our psyche and our choices too.

47

Beware of theses influences and how it affects your choice of in health, beauty and wellness.

Adopting good daily habits such as exercise, stretching, deep breathing, and meditation will positively influence your body, mind, spirit, and your skin health.

➤ **Harsh weather:** Extreme cold and extreme hot will tax your skin. Cold weather can crack skin and the damage could lead to infection and leave scars. Hot weather can cause dry skin and minor disorders such as itches and acne.

➤ **Lack of proper care of the skin:**

Not cleaning the skin properly by leaving dirt and toxins in the pores can cause many problems for the skin besides acne.

Public facilities in bus, airplanes, and stores without proper precautions could result in the contract of bacteria, viruses and diseases.

Herpes, genital warts, and other venereal diseases can be transmitted from sexual intercourse.

Fecal residues in the anus could cause itching and a feeling of dirtiness.

Use herbal essential oil spray to clean your private parts after using the bathroom or having sex. Silver Shield Gel of NSP is great for these purposes.

Women should always wipe from front to back; men should clean their private part with clean tissues after using the bathroom.

After bath or shower, clean genitals with clean paper tissues instead of using the towel.

> **Toxins in skin care products—choosing the wrong products:**

The skin care products you choose will affect your skin's condition. Products filled with harsh chemicals can damage your skin faster so choose carefully.

If your skin is oily, using creams or moisturizers with too many ointments is not a good idea.

You shouldn't use strong cleaners and harsh soaps if you have dry and sensitive skin.

TOXINS in household cleaners, air fresheners, bleach, lye, detergent, dishwashing liquid, bug spray, furniture polish, artificial fluoride in water and toothpaste, carpet cleaner, drain cleaning products and more...

Beware of the effects of these harmful chemicals when there are times we need to use these products: Wear gloves, open windows, do not inhale the fumes.

1) Intrinsic (Internal) Skin Aging

> **Nutrition deficiency (Malnutrition):**

One of the major issues in nutrition deficiency is that people do not take herbal and natural medicines in large enough doses to help with the problem or long enough to have a lasting effect on their health.

Malnutrition occurs by not having enough nutrients for the body to neutralize, convert, transport, and eliminate toxins on the daily basis. The body is taking whatever is available in the body to try to survive, eventually depleting all the resources to function healthily. Liver function is associated directly with skin health. [22]

Eat whole foods daily. We need good proteins (250 g), good fats (4-5 tablespoon), fresh raw vegetables (3 cups), fresh fruit (1 portion), and clean water.

Drink water in small portions throughout the day, not drowning yourself in the large quantity of water, as only the first 4 ounces will go to the cells; the rest will wash out along with *minerals.*

While bottled water is readily available, we can sometimes drink less water than we need. Make sure you have an alternative resource of water at home. Faucet filters can aid in this. Put a tiny dash of Himalayan or NSP sea salt or a drop of essential oil in the filter container to disinfect the water.

---

[22] https://www.liverdoctor.com/your-skin-reflects-your-liver/

The IN.FORM daily meal plan is shown here:

DAILY MEAL PLAN

CATERGORY	TOTAL DAILY SERVINGS	SERVING SIZE
Meal Protein	3	Palm Size
Snack Protein	2	1/2 Palm Size
Vegetables	6	1/2 - 1 cup
Fresh Greens	5 ounces	Varies
Fruit	1	Varies
Legumes (optional)	1	½ cup
Dairy (optional)	1	Varies
Oils/Fats	5	Varies
Water	Half of your body weight in ounces	Up to 100 ounces

IN.FORM
EMPOWERED TO TRANSFORM

NATURES SUNSHINE

Water structure can easily change. Do not leave plastic bottles of water in the car or hot area or reuse the bottle. Also, saliva can contaminate the water. [23]

> ### Inability to digest food and water (need enzymes):

We eat and drink daily, yet in many ways, our body cannot digest the foods we eat or absorb the water we drink; therefore, our body can't bring proper nutrients to the cells to help them regenerate.

---

[23] https://www.banthebottle.net/articles/7-bottled-water-myths-busted/

➤ Vitamins, minerals, and trace minerals deficiency:

Our body needs vitamins and trace minerals to stay healthy and grow. Most of the vitamins we need our body can't make, so we need to take them from foods and the sun.

The discussion between synthetic and natural vitamins continues for decades. In our opinion, your body is a biological system—it can't easily digest synthetic and petroleum products.

In fact, sometimes it treats them as toxins if it can't get rid of them. It stores them inside, causing reactions by the organs such as allergies and illnesses.

Nature's Sunshine, Pure Herbs, Dr. Terry and Doc D. herbs are my main sources of vitamins and herbal products. In my opinion, it makes total sense to use best natural resources to provide good nutrients for my skin and body.

➤ Toxins inside that your body can't get rid of:

In modern society, digestive issues are one of the most common problems. With so many processed foods that lack fiber and water, foods stay in the stomach and large intestines longer and ferment, causing gas, bloating, indigestion, even infection, and illnesses.

The inability to sweat also causes the body to retain toxins, which damage the organs and skin.

Constipation means there are toxins in the guts. Foods fermenting inside your body and coating the large intestine with thick paste create a breeding ground for candida, yeast, and bacteria.

Over a period of time, these toxins can leak back into the small intestine, get inside the blood, and contaminate the whole body. This is referred to as Leaky Gut Syndrome.[24]

➤ Hormone imbalance:

Changes in your body can tremendously influence the skin. The menstrual cycle in women can cause drastic skin changes. Pregnancy and menopause also affect the skin.

The testosterone hormone in men also affects mood, sexual performance, and overall health.

The endocrine system is the composition of the pineal gland, pituitary gland, pancreas, ovaries, testes, thyroid gland, parathyroid gland, hypothalamus, gastrointestinal tract, and adrenal glands. It produces many kinds of hormones needed for different body functions.

The Metabolic system breaks foods down to provide energy for the body. The thyroid gland produces T3 and T4 hormones that help control metabolism.[25]

- The pancreas produces insulin boosting sugar go from blood to the cells, where it can be used as energy.
- Pituitary gland or Master gland is the major gland in the hormone system.
- The adrenal glands produce cortisol. It is the stress-response hormone, the flight-or-fight hormone. It is a life-sustaining steroid chemical needed to alert a human of a potentially dangerous situation.

---

[24] http://guthealthproject.com/leaky-gut-syndrome-effects-health/
[25] https://forums.t-nation.com/t/hormones-and-health/211488

- However, too much cortisol for an extended period can cause adrenal fatigue, weight gain, high blood pressure, ulcers and more.

Signs of imbalance in hormones include weight gain, digestion issues, insomnia, cravings, belly fat, and muscle loss.

Changing eating habits such as eliminating gluten, sugar, and wheat and eating organic foods with natural plant enzymes and fibers can help regain hormone balance.

Also, take proper dietary supplements to help the body regain and retain its hormone balance.

> **Telomeres shortening:**

Telomeres are the caps on each DNA strand. They protect chromosomes from sticking to each other, and they affect how cells age. They are like the caps of your shoestrings, safeguard the strings from damage and getting frayed.

The telomeres get shorter with age and stress, when this happens, the cells can't function properly in various systems, like the immune system, causing diseases and premature aging.

One of the supplements that can be beneficial for the skin is Fiber Blast Growth Factor. Nature's Sunshine's Astragalus could help the telomeres. [26]

Another product of Nature's Sunshine for men and women to fight aging and the age-related deterioration process is DHEA-F for women and DHEA-M. [27]

---

[26]   http://renegadehealth.com/blog/2015/02/20/5-reasons-to-add-astragalus-to-your-anti-aging-supplement-plan

> **Various inherited, inherited genes and medical conditions:**

Some of the rare skin diseases like: Epidermolysis bullosa, Darier's Disease, Dystrophic Epidermolysis Bullosa are inherited skin diseases. [28]

Illnesses such as autoimmune system disease can cause malnutrition, hives, rashes, and make your skin lose its firmness and elasticity. This can cause thinning, and prevent you from sweating which provides proper cooling and helps rid the body of toxins.

Allergies and other breathing disorders can result in insufficient oxygen to nourish the cells.

> **Sleep deprivation:**

Sleep is important for us. It is a natural thing. Each person has different sleeping needs; nevertheless, if you lack sufficient rest and sleep, it will affect your skin and your performance.

2) The Silent, Invisible Killers

The most dangerous factors of skin disorders are invisible. They include stress, self-sabotage, self-punishment, self-hate, disrespecting your body and life, unhappiness, despair, hopelessness, emotional disturbances, blockages, shocks, traumas, myths, mental illnesses, negative beliefs, tragedy attachments, and spiritual homelessness.

---

[27] http://theyouthdoctor.com/?sn=4200-7

[28]

http://www.britishskinfoundation.org.uk/SkinInformation/AtoZofSkinDisease.aspx

> **Unhappiness, despair, hopeless:** Not knowing how to bring your energy back to healthy level will affect all of your systems. Laughing alone is one of the best free natural medicines a person has → **Did you laugh today?**

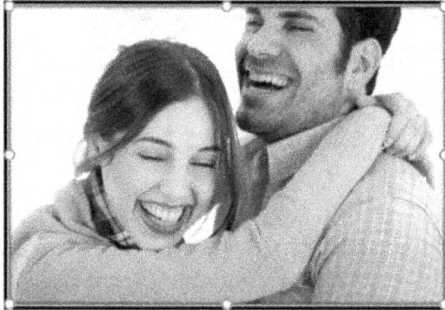

It has been medically been proven that laughter is an effective pain killer.

Image courtesy of photostock / FreeDigitalPhotos.net

> **Stress** is the worry that something bad is going to happen in the future. Stress puts pressure on the brain to try to cope with it, producing cortisol. Accumulation of cortisol has devastating effects on your skin, causing flare-ups, allergies, skin disorders, and more.

➢ **Mental unresolved issues:** Issues concerning family, money, relationships, cultures, information, and other issues can result in interpersonal conflicts. The mind is confused over the functions and values of the person and the unclear influences of the beliefs. We believe this is the root cause of many mental diseases such as Lupus and other autoimmune system problems. Left alone, the brain and body will heal itself. With conflicting thoughts, the body becomes confused and can produce unhealthy cells.

➢ **Emotional, shock, cellular level traumas:** Tragedies, accidents, physical hurts, and other experiences can leave permanent marks or blockages in your subconscious and become your beliefs and habits without you recognizing it.

They can control most of your behavior—as much as 90%. Recognize and try to replace them with new, happy beliefs.

➤ **Spiritual homelessness (being unaware of the dignified, honored human being part of you):**

Lack of self-love, self-respect, self-nurturing; self-sabotage, self-punishment, negative beliefs, and traumas contribute to stress, worries, and fears.

Unless these are addressed and healed, your skin and your body will continue to be under attack every second of the day!

FORGIVE & FORGET & CLARITY: CRUCIAL IN HEALING

Lift the shame (guilt) of immorality, unethical acts

Heal the hurt (open invisible wound of the heart)

> ➤ Clean the pain (physical imbalance)
> ➤ Clear the suffering (emotional freedom)
> ➤ Clarity of Good Health

FORGIVE ONESELF – FORGIVE OTHERS –
ASK FOR FORGIVENESS – LEARN TO
RELEASE THEM AND LET THEM GO AND
TO BE FREE TO BE IN TRUE, BEAUTY,

Learn Energy Healing Combined with Modern Technologies for Total Health

In the past decades, people have awakened to the idea and become more aware of the existence of the invisible energy all around human beings that can affect the well-being of a person, group, society, country, and even the world. I struggled for years to attempt to heal my physical body as a stand-alone project without taking this energy into account. Needless to say, it just didn't work.

We are energy and we have connections with the Divine and Earth. Not using this available energy that is all around us to help in healing is missing one of the most important elements of total health.

Some of these master healers who helped me release my obstacles in connecting with the energy sources include:

❖ Brent Phillips helped me to clear my traumas of several decades, from war to separation, tragedies, and sickness. I continue to use Brent's clearing traumas techniques even at the present time. These are powerful, timeless and effective procedures.
Combining with learning from the Divine and connect with Earth in Healing H.A.P.P.Y. Bubbles Systems, I now have the freedom to pursue my passions and create my reality the way I desired.
Brent's life-changing services is here: **theformulaformiracles.com**

❖ Daniel the Healer provides psychic surgery to remove curses, blocks, and connect me back to my Life Force. See **Danielthehealer.com**

❖ Dr. Karl Wolf of Movement Feedback goes to the quantum field and reads your *myths* (myths are the beliefs, the stories you have in your subconscious) and shows you how to clear them. I do not fully understand it, yet it works for me beautifully. **www.karlwolfe.com**

❖ Spiritual Being, friends of humans; see **Lazaris.com**

❖ Dr. Paul Scheele of Learning Strategies. The first audio I bought after my car accident was *You Deserve It!* Yes, it worked! See also the *Photo-Reading, Genius Code, 4 Powers for Greatness*. Wonderful resources.

Chapter 3: Factors Affecting Skin Health—Summary Box

1. External: Your skin is a sponge for toxic household chemicals, harmful sun rays, and harsh weather. Lack of proper skin care, lifestyle habits of drinking and smoking, emotional, social influences, all contribute to skin disorders and can be easily avoidable.

2. Learn to read UPC codes for potentially harmful chemicals and GMO products. First number 9 on the label indicates an organically grown product.

3. The origin of goods and radiation processes when imported into your country could eliminate the values in foods, skin and hair products.

4. Internal: These include aging, the inability to digest food and water, vitamin deficiency, toxins in the body, hormone imbalance, pH imbalance, various medical conditions, sleep deprivation. Don't forget to care for your brain (your personal bio-computer) too.

5. Invisible killers: Emotional stress, self-sabotage, self-punishment, negative beliefs, traumas, self-hate, disrespect of the Self, being SELF and life, depression, are all important *negative* factors in skin health.

6. Combined modern technologies with Earth & Divine Intelligence:
   a. Continue to check up with your medical doctors, dentists, chiropractors, pharmacists.
   b. Learn muscle testing, Magical Scanner to find and confirm the products for your skin needs.
   c. Use herbal, natural, quality products
   d. Harmonize and balance your physical with divinity energies sources.

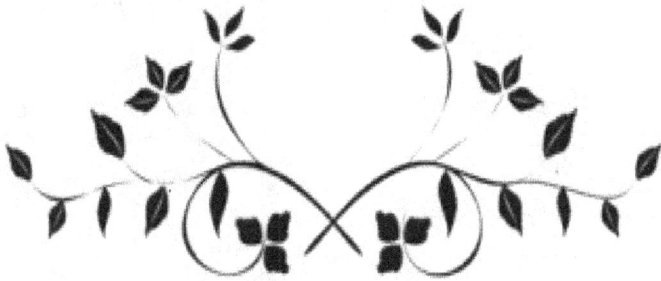

This page intentionally left blank.

Chapter 4 —The Tools: Not Rocket Science!

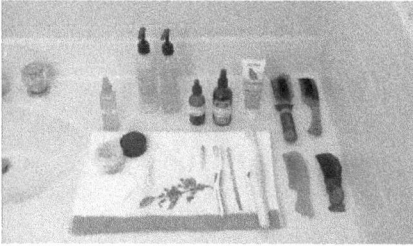

Face-Cleaner Brush, Hair Brush, Body Brush & Combs

Brushes come into contact with your pores, as well as a variety of other essential parts of your skin's anatomy. As such, you have to be careful about which types of brushes you use, and how you use them.

Brushes have different effects when used on different skin types or parts of your body, and help to clean out the dead cells.

Keep brushes and combs clean with water and soap or baking soda.

Do not over brush to avoid irritation.

Test bristle or plastic brushes to find what is best for you.

Never brush wet hair to prevent breakage.

Use organic products to color your hair to prevent toxin buildup.

Use organic natural, herbal, essential oils, creams, and lotions for your face and body.

Use rounded end for hair brushes

and a natural fiber for face brush whenever possible. Choose a wide tooth comb for easy hair combing, especially when your hair is wet. In Asia, ornate buffalo horn combs are very popular. They have no static, are beautiful, and very efficient in massaging the scalp.

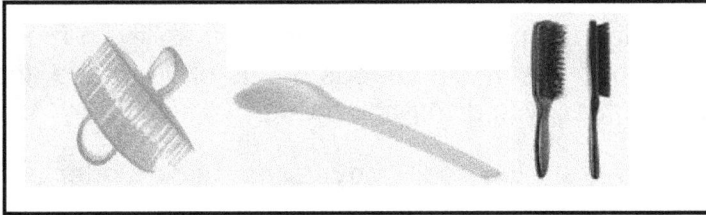

> **Toothbrush & toothpaste**

We love electric toothbrushes. They are convenient and effective in preventing cavities. Use a tongue cleaner to clean bacteria on your tongue and eliminate bad breath.

In Asia, specifically in Vietnam, we use tongue cleaners from a very early age. Your tongue collects a lot of things throughout the day. You eat, you drink, and breathe how many times a day? You have mucus from your nose. All of which come into contact with your tongue. We think using a tongue cleaner helps greatly for your overall health.

Quite a few supermarkets now are selling tongue cleaners. We highly recommend you pick some up next time you go to the store. They're very simple to use. You just bend the cleaning tool and then scrape your tongue with it. Then you rinse or clean the device with soap and water, organic vinegar apple cider, or Super Group spray.

For toothpaste: We choose a natural one without the harmful chemical fluoride; the inside of your mouth is very sensitive, so why take the chance?

➤ **Hands, Fingers, Feet, Body, Sounds, Thoughts & Praying**

Yes, these tools are awesome and absolutely free. Another bonus is that they are easily accessible. You can massage on the bus and the train quietly, and enjoy the relaxation anywhere and at any time.

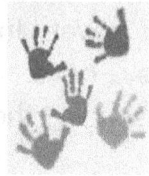

The hands and fingers give you the ability to massage or use acupressure on various points of your face and body; sometimes with discretion though.

You can stretch your body, arms, neck, under arms, and facial muscles.

You can create sounds that will help to calm your mind and take in breaths that will heal any emotional stress that you may be having. ☺

Note: Healing sounds 528 HZ is a great program for DNA repair and miracles.

Praying is talking to God. You can pray or smile—both of those are incredibly useful and free of charge. Praying comes in many forms: from simple asking God or the Universe (or whatever name you use for the Higher Power) to help healing your ailments.

You can say the "Blessings", or you can do a "Detach" action that allows you to ascend above your physical being temporarily. As for smiling, it can help your body to create a chemical called melatonin. Melatonin is the 'Happiness" chemical!

There's a quote by Mother Teresa that I've always thought was very profound- *"Peace begins with a smile."* That's entirely true.

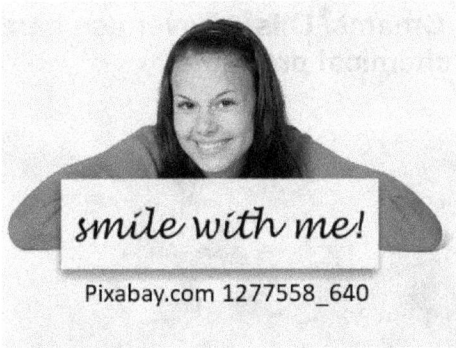

smile with me!

Pixabay.com 1277558_640

Smiling can work miracles. Your facial muscles are connected to your brain, and giving a smile is one of the best ways to show your emotions.

Expressions can also give you the power to show happiness, sadness, and sickness, and your brain will react to these emotions accordingly.

The next time that you feel rushed or stressed out, instead of thinking of how much stress you are under, change your perception and your thought. Maybe you can say this:

"I am going to enjoy this day of mine no matter what" and smile.

I have found it extremely helpful to pray and ask for help when I feel like I am rushing around in life. Just stop time and remind yourself that you don't have to be like the White Rabbit in Wonderland. Then smile, and realize that right now, at this very moment, you can surround yourself with joy and calm.

> ➢ **Soaps, Creams, Oils – Never use harsh chemical products**

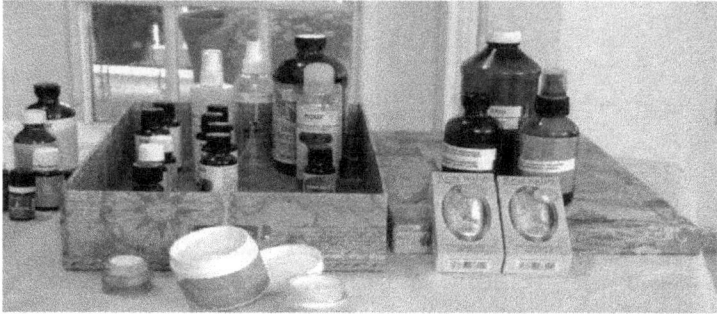

We are a fantastic example of biology in action. Our organic bodies cannot process chemical, synthetic materials, and other ingredients. In fact, some of the chemicals and synthetic elements that are found in beauty care products today are poisonous to our bodies. Therefore, as a matter of fact, they could do more harm than good.

Our skin and hair also collect bacteria and germs throughout the day. Radiation, thanks to environmental pollutants and UV rays, is another issue we have to deal with in our modern society. You can add salt (Himalayan salt or kosher salt) and organic baking soda to your bath to reduce the amount radiation in your skin.

So, if we don't want to use chemical-filled products that are found on store shelves today, what kind of creams and oils should we be using to cleanse and nourish our skin, body, face, and hair? Well, a great alternative is products that are pH balanced, particularly those that don't contain any radical elements.

The skin on the outside of your body has a natural pH balance of 5.5, slightly acidic. When this surface layer is in equilibrium, it will be relaxed and won't be prone to dry out, crack easily, and, aside from winkles forming, be susceptible to sun damage. (or cry out, for that matter, for moisturizer.)

The best soap for face and body I found is the Nu-Skin Clean bar[29].

Organic Apple Cider Vinegar is one of the most amazingly and versatile pH balancing products that I have come across. Best of all, it is inexpensive and helps to clean away bacteria and germs from your skin. Virgin (cold pressed) or unprocessed coconut oil is also great for the skin, mainly because it absorbs easily and boosts your skin's fatty nutrition content.

Essential oils are also well-liked and ideal for body and skin health. In fact, I have become "addicted" to them. I love using these because they can be applied topically, given that they, too, quickly absorb into your skin. It can also clean and clear the odor in the room very fast.

29

https://www.nuskin.com/content/nuskin/en_US/products/shop/donate/621103
54.html

A blend of equal portions of cedar wood, rosemary, lavender, and sage is traditionally believed to help with hair loss, baldness, and dandruff. Apply on your hair before bedtime or in the morning.

Rosemary, lavender, cypress, and thyme may likewise help a man's beard to grow. Biotin and sulfurzyme can support normal hair growth.

Tea Tree oil is amazing to quickly heal insect bites and fix irritation on the skin.

> *Be sure to test the organic oils before using to avoid allergic reactions.*

> *Keep oil, hair, and facial products out of reach of children.*

> ### "Super-Group" Secret Healing Water Composite

This wonderful blend is easy to make; and has several daily usages:
  - Refresh hair, skin, face, body, underarm et al.
  - Clean body: ears. nose, mouth, sexual organs, and butts of bacteria, harmful radiation, viruses, chemicals, and parasites.
  - Refresh bed, pillows, linen, and clothes.
  - Clean desk, tables, bathroom, etc.
  - Clean public seat, toilet seat in train, bus, or airplane.

Super-Group Denville NJ Healing Water Recipe:

18-20 oz. of filtered water or
Nature's Sunshine Nature's Fresh Enzymes Spray (if using Enzymes, just add essential oils).

2 -4 oz. organic apple vinegar cider,
99 grains of Himalayan salt or sea salt (just kidding: a tiny touch to improve absorption, is ok).

7-14 drops of essential oil – sage or lavender.

7-14 drops of essential oil – rosemary or peppermint.

7-14 drops of essential oil – Inspire or anything else you like.

➔ Add unlimited of Healing H.A.P.P.Y. Bubbles blessings!

➢ **Silver Shield Gel** [30]

Silver Shield has 20 parts-per-million (ppm) of pure silver nanoparticles in a topical gel. (US Patent 7,135,195). This product is non-toxic and poses no risk of heavy metal contamination, and it provides a broad-spectrum immune support.

Silver is prominent in traditional medicine. It has potent antibacterial properties and can fight infections, control food spoilage, and purify drinking water.

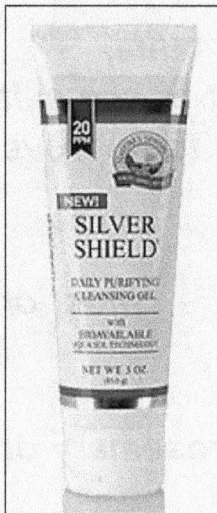

We, Doc D. and Super-Group, love Silver-Shield products and have them readily available in our first-aid kit! We use them for disinfecting cuts, insect bites, face cleaner, food poisoning, and more.

➢ **Other Private Label Creams of Doc D. & Uncle Al – not available anywhere else:**
  ➢ N-Max: Nerve Cream
  ➢ Facelift
  ➢ S.C.R.T.R: remove Scars
  ➢ Dissolve: dissolve crystals at knuckles

➢ Varicose veins
➢ And many others…

The special thing about these creams is the herb percentage put in the lotion. Usually there is 10-15%; Uncle Al puts in 35%-40%. Please visit: **FunHappyStore.com** for more information

---

[30] http://theyouthdoctor.com/?sn=4952-8

> **Exercise & Massage & Stretching – This book and the demonstration DVD focus on Head & Face (please see the appropriate chapters)**

All these tools are used to achieve the common goal of harmonizing, balancing, and generating energies for your living fitness. Select a system or a combination of methods to do daily in bed before you get up and before sleeping will help to maintain your health status.

Exercise is not only good for weight loss, but it is also an essential part of body detoxification. Ideally, you should include cardiovascular exercises in your workout routine as they will help you to sweat our impurities. Yoga is also rated high, given that it gives you the chance to eliminate stress. Stress is also a form of toxicity to our bodies. Exercising will enable you to reduce your stress levels, regardless of where the pressure is coming from (i.e. work, home, and relationships).

Do not forget to take vitamins and trace minerals, though, because your body will need them more when you sweat and exercise.

Though it's probably common sense, it's worth mentioning all the same: you should avoid smoking, taking drugs, or drinking alcohol if you want to eliminate toxins.

Once you begin the naturally cleansing process, you'll probably find that it becomes a way of life. You will notice that you are looking and feeling better and that it's not challenging whatsoever to keep up the good work.

Try and you will feel magnificent! Your body will love you and thank you!

Chapter 4: The Tools: Not Rocket Science—Summary Box

1. Know the tools: Protect your skin against external factors, internal factors, and unseen harmful sources.

2. Avoid common skin issues by understanding your skin's needs:
   a. Proper nutrition (bless the food you eat, enjoy), proper waste elimination.
   b. Clean air (learn deep breathing and make it a habit)
   c. Clean water (bless the water you drink, don't be stingy because water costs money. Find effective resources—filters and faucet filters)
   d. Love yourself (be happy)

3. Your skin is part of your body and your being. Take good care of it—it is a fun thing to do. Take vitamins, supplements.

4. Use organic, natural products. Maintain a pH 5.5. Explore new products once in a while and be selective.

5. Know what type of skin you have to choose the proper products for your skin type.

6. Pay attention to your face and skin for any issues,

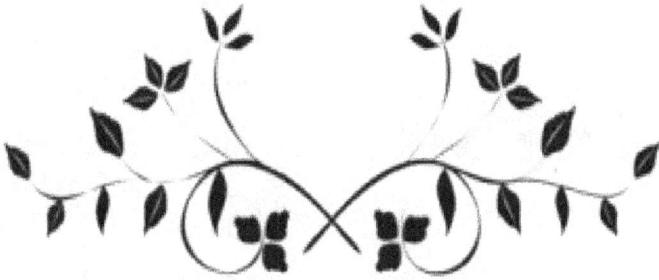

This page intentionally left blank.

Chapter 5—Facial Skin Tests

Skin Types

Care for the Face

Sagging Muscles*: The older we get, the 43-60 muscles on the face get weaker, and pull down the entire face. Correct this by:*

❖   *Exercising Your Face*
❖   *Acupressure*

Aging Skin: *Wrinkles, Age Spots, and Dryness*

❖   *Use Creams, Oils*
❖   *Massage*
❖   *Brush*

Aging Cells*: Thinner skin, less plump, and not so smooth*

❖   *Good Nutrition*
❖   *Dietary Supplements*
❖   *Massage*
❖   *Use Creams, Oils*
❖   *Exercise*
❖   *Acupressure*

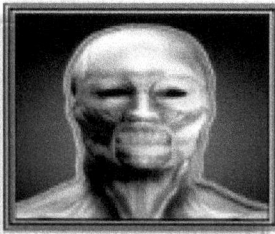

The **face** is a central sense organ complex, normally on the ventral surface of the head for animals that have one.

It can, depending on the definition and in the human case, include the hair, forehead, eyebrow, eyelashes, eyes, nose, ears, cheeks, mouth, lips, philtrum, temple, teeth, skin, and chin.

The face is used for expression, appearance, and identity among other things. It also has the senses of olfaction, taste, hearing, and vision.[31]

---

[31] http://en.wikipedia.org/wiki/Face

Toxicity: *Biochemical changes can damage cells and tissues, resulting in slower healing or permanent damage.*

* ❖ **Proper Nutrition**
* ❖ *Drink Water – ½ of your weight up to 100 oz*
* ❖ *Stop Smoking*
* ❖ *Avoid Alcohol*
* ❖ *Detoxify*
* ❖ *Practice Prevention*
* ❖ *Exercise*
* ❖ *Avoid Exposure to Extreme Weather*
* ❖ *Relax*
* ❖ **Do Not Stress**
* ❖ **Get Enough Sleep**

Let your face be The Ambassador of Your Being. Your face is the reflection of your inner physical and emotional health.

o Take good care of your whole body with the proper nutrition and water, which will help the skin on your face.

o Smile to avoid stress as well as negative emotions. *When you have negative feelings or emotions, simply send them out to the universe with 10,000 blessings. This so the negative energies can be transformed into good blessing energies, harming no one. Recycle good thoughts.*

o Pay attention to what your skin needs; adjust your routine for the best results.

Simple Skin Tests

The purpose of these tests is to learn more about your skin type and its conditions so that you can repair it.

1. **Your Past, Present, and Future Face (Muscle-Sagging Test)**
   1. **Face**
      a) **Take a mirror, look up**: this is how you looked 5 years ago.
      b) **Look straight:** this is how you look now.
      c) **Look down:** this is how you are going to look 5 years from now.
      d) With age, muscles start to sag. If the muscles on your face feel like they are falling off your face, then you have a muscle-sagging issue.
      e) Laugh lines are wrinkles on the lower face.
      f) Look at the corners of your mouth, are they curving down?
      g) How are your eyes? Do you have: double vision, tired eyes, bags under your eyes, drooping eyes?
      h) Look at your neck. Do you have extra skin forming wrinkles there? Do you have double chin? Do the veins under your neck show and are they pronounced? Are you straining?

```
           MUSCLE SAGGING REMEDIES
➢ Supplements and Natural fat and Select Creams and Oils:
  Collartrim  from  NSP:  Facelift  in  an  herbal  bottle!
  (FunHappyStore.com)
➢ Massage  cellulites  with  Dissolve  cream  (Doc  D  and
  Uncle Al)
➢ Face & Eyes exercise, massage, acupressure points
➢ Remove dead cells and Increase muscle tones
➢ Add 7 drops of Frankincense Oil in Uncle Al Facelift Cream
  (FunHappyStore.com)
```

2. Body & Arms & Legs & Elbows & Knees & Ankles

a)   How do the muscles under your skin feel? Do you
have cellulite?[32] Are your muscles firm and soft and full
of energy, or weak, creaky, or squishy and squashy?

b)   Are there cellulites on your belly, under your arms,
or between your legs?

c)   Are you overweight?

d)   How are your hands, fingernails?

e)   How are your knees?

f)   How are your ankles? Do they squeak when you
move your feet or walking?

```
           JOINTS AND MUSCLES
➢ Supplements:  Calcium, manganese, silica and
  Natural fat %.
➢ Exercise, massage, acupressure points.
➢ Stretch or jump on the trampoline to increase joint
  flexibility.
```

---

[32] Cellulite is fat under the skin. Cellulitis is the bacterial infection under the
skin.

2) "Inside Skin Test." And Sexual Organs

    a) Is it itching?

    b) Look at your sexual organ or gently feel it. Do you feel bumps, warts, or herpes sores?

    c) Feel your anus; is there a bulb there, as in **hemorrhoids**?

INSIDE SKIN REMEDIES

➤ "Super-Group Healing water" & Selected Creams & Oils

➤ Exercise, massage, acupressure points

➤ Supplements & Protein & Natural fat & Radiation Cleanse, Parasite Cleanse.

➤ Uncle Al herb creams: for hemorrhoids, Brain Storm cream in **'FunHappyStore.com'**

➤ Use Healing H.A.P.P.Y Bubbles Systems™: **"The Eternal Youth Methods"** to clean radiations, parasites, harmful chemicals,

---

3) Skin Tent Test (Elasticity Test)
(Losing elasticity of the skin can be caused by aging, a nutrition deficiency, or an inability to digest fat).

    a) Take your thumb and index fingers, gently pin the skin on top of your hand, hold for a few seconds.

    b) If your skin forms a tent, see how long it takes the skin to flatten. The longer it takes, the more your skin lacks elasticity.

```
┌─────────────────────────────────────────┐
│          ELASTICITY FOR SKIN             │
│   ➢ Super Group Healing water & Selected │
│     Creams & Oils for skin type.         │
│   ➢ Exercise, massage, acupressure       │
│     points.                              │
│   ➢ Supplements & Protein & Natural Fat  │
└─────────────────────────────────────────┘
```

4) Skin Type Test

There are five types of skin (and different treatment options that you should use, depending upon your particular skin type):

a) **Normal skin:** Normal skin has no trace of oil on skin, skin relaxes and no acne or flakes (it may have a few blemishes).
   - Use gentle products to cleanse your skin.
   - Tone skin with organic toner.
   - Use a mixture of essential oil and filtered water to hydrate your skin.

b) **Dry skin:** Dry skin feels dry, taut and flaky. It maybe from inherited genes. The tone of your skin is shallow, and you have tight pores. Dry skin can age prematurely and becomes easily irritated.

   Use oil based products to clean your skin
   - Keep your skin pH balanced with natural, organic toner.
   - Apply oil-based lotions or creams.
   - Use a mixture of essential oil and filtered water to hydrate your skin.
   - Don't irritate your skin any further by picking at the rough patches.
   - Don't over brush or over exfoliate your skin.
   - Use Oil-based make-up and products to prevent moisture loss.

❖ Psoriasis (Essential oils could help: Lavender, Tea Tree Oil, Frankincense, thyme, rose, coconut oil).
❖ Eczemas (fungus yeast & candida overgrown, essential oils Frankincense).
❖ Dehydration & Allergies could cause infections.

> DRY SKIN REMEDIES
> ➢ Dry skin: dehydrate ➜increase water % and water absorption %.
> ➢ Nu Skin cleaning bar, silver shield gel.
> ➢ Do not brush on dry skin, could cause breakage, need to bring the skin back to healthy level.
> ➢ Low fat & low protein in skin layers and mucous membrane ➜ Supplements & Increase Protein % and Natural Fat %.
> ➢ Gentle massage & face exercise, tapping

c) **Oily skin** types typically have large pores on the face, especially on the sides of the nose; acne (white or blackheads); and blemishes, and scars. If you have oily skin, then it's probably thick, coarse and shiny (due to excess oils).
- Use gentle, water-based products to clean your skin.
- Cleanse your pores with Apple Cider Vinegar (for pH balance).
- Do not pick at your acne or blemishes.
- Exfoliate your skin regularly.
- Use water based make-up and products.
- In the morning, be sure to clean away the sebum created in the night on your skin. Sebum is nature's way of keeping your skin hydrated, but too much can clog your pores, resulting in blemishes. Try to use gentle cleansing lotion in the morning.
- Use an organic scrub once or twice a week.

OILY SKIN REMEDIES

- ➤ Oily skin: exceed sebum, imbalance hormone, clogged pores ➔ Clean pores, spray with Super Group Healing Water. Nu-skin cleaning bar and Nu-skin Facial Spa to rid of dead cells.
- ➤ Balance hormones ➔ Supplements and Natural Protein % and Natural Fat % and Cleaning guts.
- ➤ Change to natural oil like Jojoba oil, stop commercial moisturizer.

d) **Combination skin** may be normal or dry on your cheeks, but oily in the T-Zone area (your nose and chin). Often, those with combination skin will develop acne in the crease of your nose as a result of excess oil. Use mild products that do not strip away too much acid from your skin.

- Use appropriate products for dry skin and oily skin.
- Avoid touching your face and don't pick at it.
- Exfoliate the oily skin areas.
- Use a combination of oily and dry skin products.

e) **Sensitive skin:** is very tight and easily inflamed. It can become red and itchy from a reaction to chemicals and, allergies. Redness, irritation from the sun and household cleaning products can also contribute.

- pH balances your skin.
- Use Silver Shield to kill any bacteria.
- Use organic products and a mixture of essential oils and water to hydrate your skin.
- Read labels and test products on skin before you buy, because the minerals in products could make your skin break out.

SENSITIVE SKIN REMEDIES
- Sensitive skin: low immune system, imbalance hormone → spray with Super Group Healing Water. Nerve cream and Nu Skin clean bar.
- Increase immune system – Silver Shield Gel.
- Change to natural herbal products, sunscreen to protect skin.
- Pay attention to household cleaners that could cause allergy reactions.
- Supplements (Krill Oil, Omega blend) and Natural Protein % and Natural Fat % and Vegetable Fruits
- Face & neck gentle massage & exercise and acupressure points.

5) Cell-Aging Test (can be caused by aging, illnesses, and the inability of the body to regenerate new cells)

a) Have a close look at your face, under your eyes, on your forearms, and the skin on your legs and check for blemishes, age spots, and varicose veins.

b) If your skin is thin and transparent, showing veins under it, your cells may be aging too fast and do not have enough nutrition to generate new cells.

c) Look at your face sideways and notice the laugh lines (*nasolabial fold*) from your nose to the mouth; are they deep?

d) Pull both your ears up; do these wrinkles disappear?

e) As we get older, the laugh lines and the mouth start to fall. This is a combination of sagging muscles and the skin losing its elasticity.

CELL-AGING SKIN REMEDIES

➤ Aging skin: low immune system, imbalance hormone ➔ spray with Super Group Healing Water. Nerve cream. Nu Skin clean bar. Silver shield gel.
➤ Increase immune system – Silver Shield Gel.
➤ Balance hormone, detox guts.
➤ Change to natural herbal products, sunscreen to protect skin.
➤ Supplements (Krill Oil, Curcumin BP, Collatrim) & Natural Protein % & Natural Fat % & Vegetable Fruits.
➤ Varicose veins ➔ Uncle Al varicose cream or Nerve cream.
➤ Face & neck gentle massage & exercise & acupressure points,

Facial Cleaning & Toning for Both Men & Women

- ❖ The goal in the morning is to clean and protect the skin for the activities of the day.

- ❖ Men have skin and hair too, and they need to know how to care for their face too. Buy this book for them, and help them!

- ❖ Drinking hot water with fresh lemon or a few drops of organic oil first thing in the morning is good for your body overall [33].

- ❖ Pay attention to the changes and improvements of your skin every day. Scrub twice a week if needed.

- ❖ Clean eyes, ears, nose, mouth, tongue, body.

- ❖ Fresh lemongrass and fresh ginger drink in the morning before coffee: nutritious and delicious, great to clean overall system.

  Do not drink coffee or green tea on an empty stomach, especially in the morning. It is too acidic for your body! You can enjoy it after breakfast.

---

[33] *110 Uses of Essential Oils* booklet

FRESH LEMONGRASS & FRESH GINGER ROOT DRINK

- ➤ Simmer for 20 minutes one stem of chopped lemongrass and one small ginger root in a small pot
  - ➤ Pour 10 ounces of this water into a large cup, mix in:
    - o 1 tablespoon of organic coconut oil
    - o 1 tablespoon of organic coconut milk
    - o ½ teaspoon of raw honey
    - o ½ teaspoon of dandelion mix (optional)

Enjoy! This would fulfill 2 portions of fat needed daily!

Take your protein shake or breakfast with vitamins then.

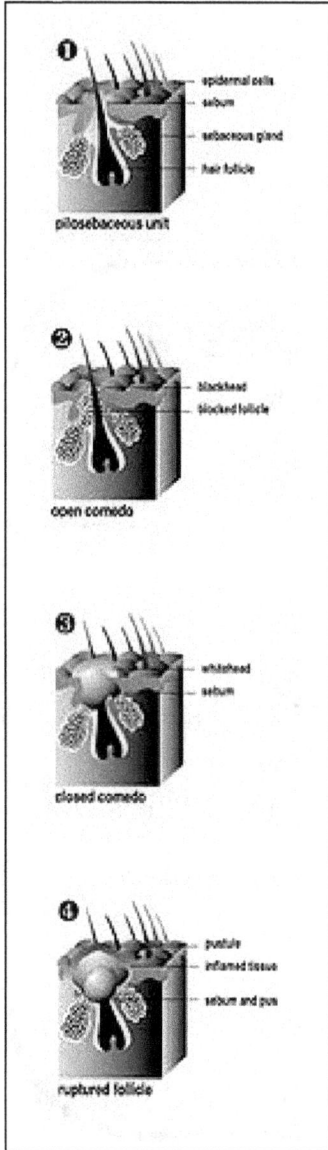

❶
- epidermal cells
- sebum
- sebaceous gland
- hair follicle

pilosebaceous unit

❷
- blackhead
- blocked follicle

open comedo

❸
- whitehead
- sebum

closed comedo

❹
- pustule
- inflamed tissue
- sebum and pus

ruptured follicle

In the morning, while you do not have to remove makeup, you still need to clean off the sebum created during the night on your skin. Sebum is nature's way of keeping your skin hydrated, but too much can clog the pores and cause blemishes. Use a gentle cleansing lotion in the morning.

1. The sebaceous glands of the skin produce an oily substance, composed of keratin, fat, and cellular debris called *sebum*. Sebum's job is to protect the skin from drying.

2. Excess sebum can clog the follicles and bacteria could growth. A blackhead or open comedo could be the resulting of this on the skin.

4. If the plug is below the skin surface, it is called a "whitehead" or "closed comedo."

5. When the sebum pocket or bacteria is too much, the follicle will rupture. It can then spill the contaminated content into the tissues around it and damage them. These damaged tissues can become a pustule cyst or an abscess. They can become infected or leave a scar on the skin.

Help your children to understand the importance of cleaning and caring for their skin!
They will thank you forever!

❖ In the evening, always remove all makeup, especially eye mascara and eyeliner, and clean your face and neck. Scrub, if needed, to exfoliate your skin. Wash your face and neck and apply toner. Using apple cider vinegar as toner could correct bad skin tone; it can control oil, antiseptic, and pH balance, and stimulate circulation. Mix ½ ounce of apple cider vinegar in 4 ounces of filtered water, adjusting the strength accordingly for your skin. Super Group Healing Water is a great alternative solution for all types of skin.

❖ Use organic scrub once or twice a week, if needed.

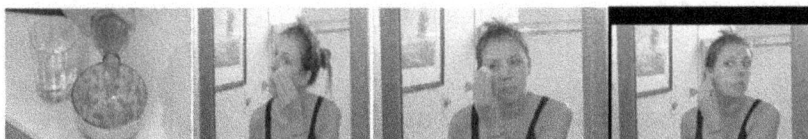

❖ **Face oils (use any combination you like)**

> Equal parts lavender, helichrysum, Gentle Baby[34], rose, frankincense, geranium, hyssop, melrose [35], rosehip, lemon, and frankincense and patchouli.

> Skin oil – Equal parts lavender, lemon, frankincense and patchouli mixed with a few ounces of lecithin oil.

> Cream – Put a few drops of your choice into a moisturizing cream, mix well.

> Scar – Equal parts helichrysum, rosemary, and lavender mixed with liquid parts lecithin. Doc D and uncle Al: Scar cream is great.

> Eyes – Equal parts of frankincense, lavender, and lemon.

---

[34] http://www.experience-essential-oils.com/gentle-baby-essential-oil.html
[35] http://www.experience-essential-oils.com/melrose-essential-oil.html

❖ Other Formulas

➢ Toner – Organic apple cider vinegar and spring water or revitalized biogenic water. (http://revitalizedbiogenic.com):1 part of apple vinegar and 10 parts of water.

➢ Organic lavender, rosemary oil, and spring water: 4 ounces of water, 7 drops of oils. Refrigerate, spray to refresh skin, hair, neck, and spine. If desired, add other oils.

➢ Create your own favorite drinks, change them once in a while

➢ Liquid chlorophyll is great for cleaning toxins out from your blood, helping your skin greatly. [36]

➢ Mix one tablespoon of organic apple vinegar cider with 5 ounces filtered water. Drink it after breakfast, lunch, or dinner. It will help your digestive system.

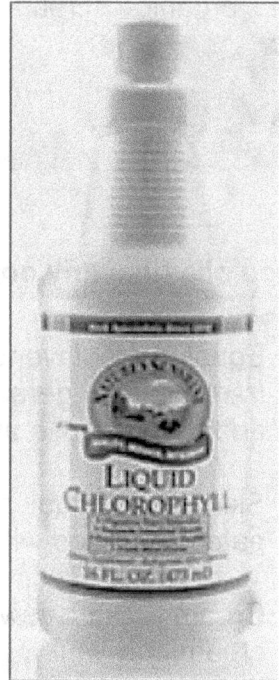

𝓢kin 𝓒are for 𝓜en

• "Men's skin care" may seem alien to some males today. However, it probably would've sounded even more alien a few years back. Men are taking care of their skin more. Hence, the markets are now flooded with male skin care

---

[36] http://theyouthdoctor.com/?sn=1683-7

products. Even though a man's skin is very different from a woman's, both skin care routines are very similar to each other.

• Much like women's skin care, men must also begin their skin care routine by cleansing their skin. Water soluble cleansers are generally the better choice. Thoroughly cleansing the skin removes the dirt, grease, and pollutants that threaten to clog the pores. Male skin is naturally oilier, which makes cleansing an important first step in your skin health regimen. You should be cleaning your skin at least once a day but preferably twice a day. However, you should try to avoid using harsh, chemical soap on your face.

• An important aspect of skin care for men is shaving. Shaving products, such as foams, gels, and creams, as well as after shave lotions, are some of the essential skin care products for men. Serious "man skin care" requires a proper selection of shaving related equipment and products. You also need to choose the right shaving tools, such as the proper razor (a swivel, flexible head is recommended).

The main thing is to know the skin type and condition. Regardless of your skin type, however, you should stay clear of alcohol-based aftershaves. Also, when you are using your razor, try to be as gentle as possible. Don't push too firmly. After all, you're trying to get rid of the hair, not the skin itself.

• The skin on a man's face is typically thicker and oilier. This is primary because males have larger pores, and their sebaceous glands are a bit more active than women's. However, moisturizers are essential, given that shaving can cause the skin to become dehydrated. After you shave, you should be applying moisturizing gels or creams. In fact, look for ones that have built-in moisturizers.

• Always use sunscreen to protect against the harmful UV radiation. As a matter of fact, a moisturizer that includes some sort of sunscreen, with vitamin B5 would be great as this will help to treat overexposure to UV rays and wind.

• When searching for the right male skin care products, opt for ones that have natural ingredients, such as Aloe Vera, sea salt, and coconut. Also, those that contain natural antiseptic oil, like lavender and tea tree, are great options.

❖ Bath Salt to Detoxify Skin – once or twice a week or when needed

1. Put 7-14 drops each of lavender, sage, frankincense, rosemary, oregano, etc. in Himalayan salt. Pour 1 tablespoon into a bathtub.
   Or just ½ cup of Epsom salt, drop in any essential oils you desire.
   Or Kosher salt, drop in any essential oils you desire
2. Put in 1/3 cup of natural baking soda.
3. Soak 5-10 minutes, head merge and hair inside the water, if desired.
4. Use natural fiber brush, soak in water and brush everything including your feet.

5. First, you will feel the water coming inside you. When you feel there are bubbles on your skin, that means the toxin inside is coming out. Stay for another 5 minutes, then start to empty the water.

Enjoy! You could make this a romantic night!

6. Rinse your hair and body with mixture of water and organic apple cider vinegar. Then rinse with clean water.
7. Dry and spray with Super Group Healing water, then apply face, body cream and massage for a few minutes.

Take a nap afterward!

Chapter 5: Facial Skin Test and Skin Types—Summary Box

There are simple skin tests for different types of skin and remedies. Know your skin needs.

    a. Hormone imbalance needs to be cared for.

    b. Low immune system needs to be looked into.

Always do your cleaning and toning first, and then exfoliate by brushing, exercising your mouth, massaging, and pulling the ears. All of these things can help eliminate wrinkles.

Facial cleaning is simple and easy to do twice daily

    a. Your body needs protein first thing in the morning.

    b. Create a simple, daily routine for twice a day, once in the morning and once in the evening.

    c. Enjoy bath salt.

Don't forget the chin and neck and hands and feet and other parts of the body.

Share the information with your family, children and friends. Help them to care for their skin health.

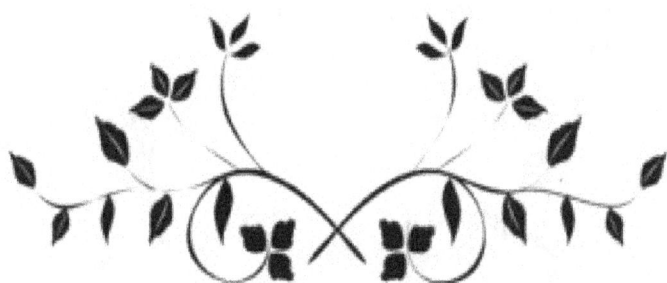

This page intentionally left blank.

Chapter 6—Remolding Your Skin: Facial Massage

After cleansing and toning, apply cream to your face:

- ➢ Avoid getting cream in the eyes.
- ➢ Massage with fingertips.
- ➢ Do twice daily, every morning and evening.

Be gentle around the eyes and neck.
Notice the feelings on your face. Stop if your skin feels irritated.

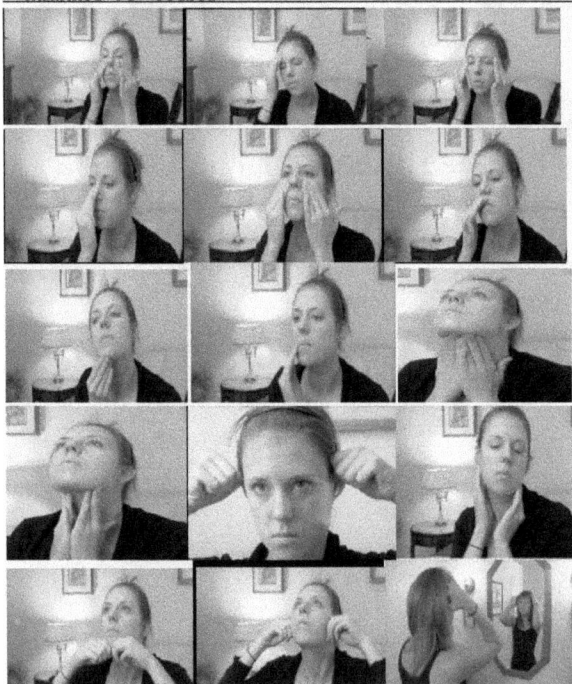

Techniques used for Massages or Brushing are the same: Muscles and skin have memories; use circular motions clockwise, then counterclockwise; this could help erase wrinkles.

Where there are deep wrinkles, e.g., eye corners & temple, gently lift or stretch the skin to massage or brush into them to remove dead cells.

You can use your fingertips or face cleaning brush to massage your face. The key is to concentrate on the area that needs attention.

Massage can help your body relax and improve circulation. It provides relief for tight muscles (knots) and other aches and pains.

It can release nerve compressions such as carpel tunnel and sciatica.

You can massage your face in any order:
❖ Start with the eyes, then the forehead, temples, nose's bridge, sides of nose, cheeks, philtrum, chin, mouth, neck, ears, behind ears, jaws.
❖ Don't forget to pull ears up and hold for a few seconds.
❖ Massage your scalp, hair, and
hairline.

Don't forget the ears!

Each ear is connected with the whole body organs inside, left and right. Massaging the ears is massaging your organs. Take one or two minutes to rub your ears daily. It increases blood flow. Breathe deeply when massaging. It is good for overall health.

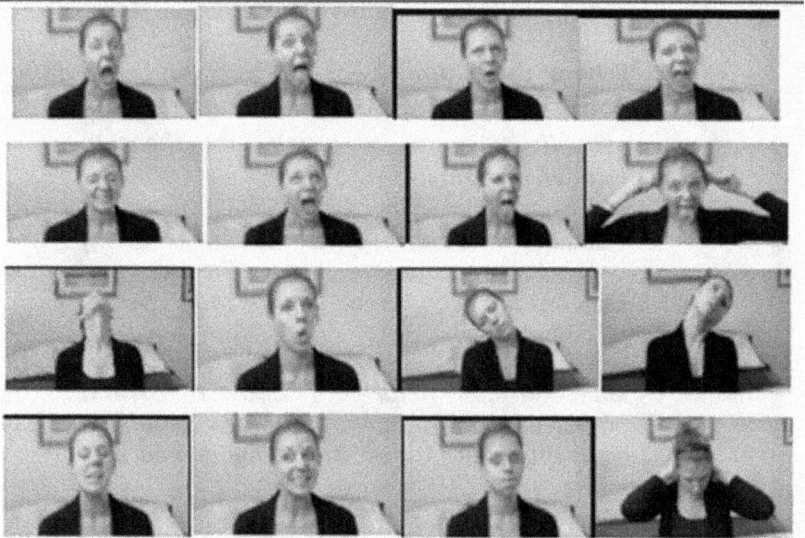

Facial Exercising

- Face exercises can be done at any point after applying face cream or oil.

- They can help relieve stress and renew energy.

- Do them anytime; combine them with massaging or brushing.

- Multitask during the day or when watching TV, exercising, cooking, etc. Doing face exercises in public might cause strong reactions from those around you, which can be hilarious and fun.

- If your skin feels tight, use tapping techniques (similar to massaging), and spray your skin with water combined with lavender/peppermint oil to relax the skin and muscles.

- Create your own exercises and have fun with them.

- Stretch every muscle on your face, release them, and stretch them again to exercise them. Make sure to exercise all the muscles—forehead, nose, cheeks, eyes, mouth, and neck—to firm them up.

- Breathe! Don't forget to breathe. Put your tongue on the roof of your mouth. Breathe in deeply through the nose, expand your stomach, hold for five counts. Breathe out slowly, through the mouth, and let the air vibrate your tongue.

ℱacial ℬrushing

❖ **Apply serum after applying cream to seal in the moisture.**

➢ Brush with the cleaning face brush once or twice a week (if desired). You can massage with fingertips if you don't want to use the brush.
➢ Can use oil instead of serum.
➢ Dip brush in lavender/peppermint water to make the brush softer.

Do not damage the first layer of the skin (epidermis); it could form a scar. Stop if your skin is feeling irritated.

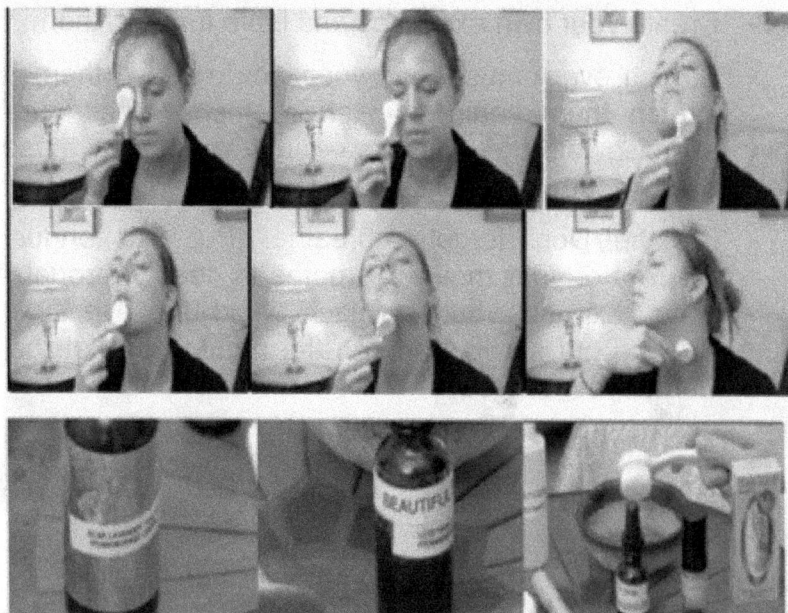

Brush in the serum and massage with cream in any order on clean face:

- ❖ *Brush clockwise and counter-clockwise 3 times. Do not over brush; it could irritate the skin.*
- ❖ *Use water with lavender; spray on the red spots; it might help.*
- ❖ *Start with the eyes, then forehead, temples, nose bridge, sides of nose, cheeks, philtrum, chin, mouth, neck, ears, behind the ears, and jaw.*
- ❖ *Brush the back of your neck and collarbone to help circulation.*

Eyes Care -Crows Feet, Eye Hoods, Bags under eyes, Eyebrow sagging (Upper eyelids)

➤ Crow's feet, which are also referred to as "smile lines," "laugh lines," and "character lines," are, unfortunately, an absolutely natural part of the aging process. As a matter of fact, just about everyone over the age of 25 will start to develop these tiny little lines or wrinkles in the corners of their eyes.

➤ Crow's feet are one of the first types of wrinkles that will start to appear and are typically caused by of years of laughing, smiling, frowning, and squinting (just think about how often you squint while looking at the computer screen). As we age, our skin begins to lose its natural elasticity. The lack of collagen and fatty acids begins to gradually diminish, and our skin's starts to lose its ability to stretch and return to its natural shape.

➤ There are a variety of other factors that reduce our skin's elasticity, as well, aside from aging. Exposure to ultraviolet light (UV) rays from the sun also results in collagen disintegration. Free radicals in the air and within the foods we eat also cause wrinkles. Even smoking can speed up the skin's aging process and make your face look older.

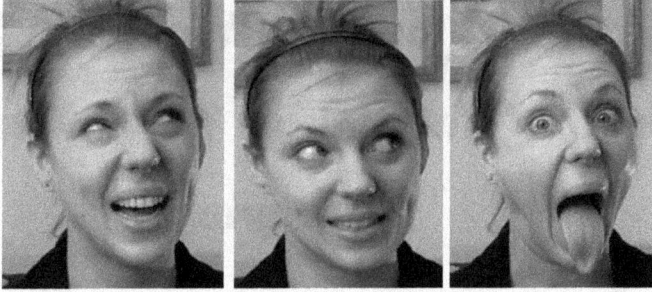

➤ The bags that develop under our eyes are caused by muscle weakness, as well as excess skin beneath the eyes. The same can lead to hoods over your eyes. Your eyebrows can also begin to sag, which is a clear indication of old age. Dark circles, on the other hand, are typically caused by illness, lack of sleep, stress, unhappiness, or fatigue.

➤ Get rid of these eyes wrinkles after you've finished cleaning and toning your skin by gently brushing, exercising or pressing acupressure points that relax the eyes. Brush gently with eyes closed both ways: clockwise and anti-clockwise on the eyelids and under the eyes. Cleaning the eyes with Rue of Liquid herb will help clean the toxins in the caterpillars of the eyes.

Nose, Mouth Wrinkles (Bunny lines, Nasolabial Wrinkles & Drooping)

Nose is important for our survival; we need it to breathe! Both sides of the nose and top of nose can accumulate acnes (white and black heads) easily. Make sure to clean daily with cleaner and brush.

Brush on and around the nose to clean the pores. Brush and massage the lines between the nose and around the mouth, called nasal labial fold lines. Exercise will also help to reduce these lines. Nu Skin spa machines definitely help!

➢ Nobody wants to show obvious signs of aging, stress, sun exposure, and gravity on their faces. When deep creases start to appear between the mouth and nose, your jaw lines grow slack and droop, and fat deposits and folds begin to appear around the neck area. You'll naturally want to get rid of them as quickly as possible. Even though they are a natural part of life, they aren't necessarily the most attractive.

➢ Wrinkles are, in essence, nothing more than a reduction of your skin's elasticity and essential fatty acids (EFT). When this occurs, your skin starts to create folds on your face. More than anything else, it is **a sign of nutrient deficiency, damage of skin layers, muscle weakness, and stress expression.**

Wrinkles on your nose are called bunny lines. If they are occurring alongside the nose and stretching to your mouth, they are called Nasolabial folds.

➢ Mouth drooping is also an unfortunate sign of aging muscle sagging. The skin on both sides of your mouth may become darker, as well, as they can be filled with dead skin cells. When cleaning your face, use a facial cleansing brush, open your mouth wide, and brush both sides of your mouth. This will help to clear away dead cells. While the philtrum is not the main factor in face lines, it's nice to tap and gently massage and exercise.

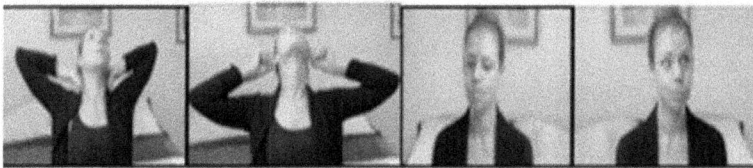

➢ Brush skin on both sides of the chin to take care of the wrinkles under the chin. Exercise the chin to get rid of a double chin.

➢ Neck wrinkles could show the age more than the face. On women, makeup helps to hide face flaws. If you want, to tell the true age of a person, look at their hands and their neck.

➤ For neck wrinkles, massage gently daily with cream, skin brush VERY lightly as the skin on the neck is very sensitive. Soft and slow exercise (not excessive to prevent the veins showing too much)

DO NOT USE ACUPRESSURE ON THE NECK

➤ A double chin is a sack of fat under the chin, and it makes it look like there is a second chin. Clean, brush, massage and exercise the mouth and neck would help to reduce the fat tissues. Tightening the skin with the Nu Skin machine definitely will help to have a younger looking neck and chin.

➤ Rub neck gently using Lymphatic detox manually massage is very helpful for your body.

➤ Find more information of "The Eternal Youth Methods" webinars for secret herbs and products to maintain youth and beautiful skin at any age on FunHappyStore.com.

Chapter 6: Facial Massage, Brushing & Exercise: Nutritional for your skin—Summary Box

1. Facial massage improves complexion and muscle tone (anti-aging).
   a. Always massage on moist skin with a spray of healing water or cream.
   b. Massage eyes gently only. Do not push on eyeballs.
   c. Massage ears and behind the ears and neck to improve the lymphatic drainage (Lymphatic system gets rid of toxins, waste. It helps the body to fight infections by carrying white blood cells to lymph nodes).

2. Facial exercise: look years younger in just 10 minutes a day. You can do it anywhere and anytime! ☺
   a. Eye exercise is great for vision and balance.
   b. Improve your expression and youthfulness.
   c. Release stress as you smile, automatically changing to happy mood.

3. The best way to reduce wrinkles is not having the them in first place! Wrinkles are caused by loss of skin elasticity, lack of muscles strength and fatty cushions in the skin. Besides exercise and massage, good nutrition and emotional happiness will help in removing them.

4. Age spots or liver spots or sun spots on face and hands can be prevented and bleached out with masques and creams and proper nutrition. DNA repair serum, Astragalus for Youth from Nature's Sunshine can help.

5. Face, eyes, nose, philtrum, chin and neck brushing: Removing dead cells and cleaning pores will:
   a. Allow new cells to grow.
   b. Improve blood circulation for easier nutrition absorption.

Chapter 7—Nails, Hair, Scalp Tests & Care

Nails, Hair and Scalp Test

1. **Nails:** Look at the nails on your hands and feet. Are they thin? cracked? brittle? Weak? Are there ridges, uneven lines? Is there fungus? Ingrown nails? How about the colors? Do they need calcium, vitamin supplements?

2. **Scalp:** Have a close look at your scalp under your hair; touch it with your fingers. Does it look dry, bumpy? Is there dandruff? Is it itchy?
Are there bald spots?

3. **Hair:** Look at your hair; is it dry, bristly, or oily? Do you have split ends?
Is your hair shiny or dull? Flexible or stiff?

Gather a handful of hair

Pull gently but firmly. Look at your hands. If you see you have a small number of loose hairs, then it may be because your follicle is not strong and your hair is falling out.

There are many reasons why hair is weak, dry, or falling out: Genetic, illness, medications, overexposure to the sun or the wind, over processed, stress, neglected, and wrong products.

A. Nail plate; B. lunula; C. root; D. sinus; E. matrix; F. nail bed; G. hyponychium; H. free margin.

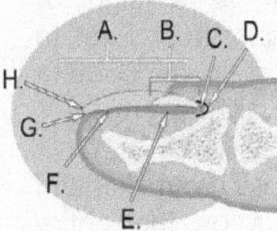

❖ Fingernails & toenails

➤ Nails need nutrition [37]

➤ Nails need to breathe and need blood to live. [38]

➤ Practice good nail hygiene: trim nails and cuticles should be gently removed.

➤ Clean underneath fingernails and toenails

➤ Excess filing, grinding and manicures can hurt nails.

➤ Spray feet and toenails with Super Group Spray or herbal water to prevent fungus and bacteria.

➤ Massage hands and nails with good herbal cream.

➤ Nails are made of non-living keratin as is hair. If nails are brittle and have deep, uneven lines, they may need calcium, manganese, and vitamin D.

➤ Some of the herbs to cure toenail fungus are: Apple Cider Vinegar, Tea Tree oil, and Orange oil.

---

[37] https://en.wikipedia.org/wiki/Nail_%28anatomy%29
[38] http://www.trendsnhealth.com/interesting-facts-about-nails/

Hair & Scalp

Hair is the barrier to protect the head from the sun and bugs and dust. Hair has two parts: the root – the follicle - and the hair shaft. The average human has about 5,000,000 hairs.

Hair growth by phases:
- ❖ 10% in the Telogen phase
- ❖ Growth phase is called Anagen
- ❖ Telogen is the resting phase, where hair stops growing and eventually falls off; new hair growth will replace it. We lose 50-100 strands of hair a day.
- ❖ Baldness is a condition where there is no hair growth to replace the hair loss.

A woman's and a man's hair are different: Usually a man loses more hair than a woman.

- ❖ Hair texture varies depend on genetics, lifestyle, and environment.
- ❖ Daily massage and brush can help.
- ❖ Nutrition for hair: pH balance, silica, krill oil, multi-vitamin.

Hair is an amazing subject

The head is exposed fully in view most of the time, except when you hide under the blanket or cover it up in the winter.

Inside the head is the brain, without it, we wouldn't be sitting here reading this book!

Outside is the scalp, on top of the scalp is the hair.

Hair is a sign of beauty from East to West in all corners of Earth.

There are millions of hairs on the entire human body; most of them are difficult to see.

While the hair on the head, including the beard (terminal hair), carries a lot of value for the desired look of the face, other hair locations such as underarm, legs, and bikini lines are removal targets to enhance smooth and desirable skin on women.

Eyelashes and eyebrows hair are also symbols of beauty.

The growth cycle of the head and beard hair varies. Hair grows from the follicle in the outer of the epidermis of the skin. This part is the root of the hair, connecting with the blood supply, providing nutrients for the new hair. The protruding part of the hair is called the shaft. As hair pushed out of the follicle, it goes through a 28 day process of Keratinization, filling the shaft with fibrous proteins. During this phase, the hair is vulnerable to dryness, and breakage, even falling out prematurely.

The Hairy Thing

Hair pH: Needs to be between 4.5 to 5.5. Chemicals will dry and damage follicles and scalp. Hair can't grow with damaged follicles.

Hair Loss (Scalp) from stress: Relax, change focus, and massage, gently brushing. Do not over brush. Wash hair every other day.

Hair Thinning: Better food, natural fat, krill oil, vitamins, and massages. Gently brush. Do not wash hair daily. Use creams and oils.

Toxicity: Detoxify, better nutrition, and prevention.

Other (Various Medical Treatments for Illnesses.)

❖ Under the scalp is the skull

Skull: The skull is the bony part of the head, which houses the brain inside and supports the face and nose. Damage to the head could cause damage to the brain and overall body functions

The scalp is the skin on the head, connecting the face and the neck. This skin is the thickest of the human body, about 8mm and has approximately about 100,000 hairs.

Scalp has five different layers: S.C.A.L.P

 ➤ S: The surface of the head which hair grows, containing numerous sebaceous glands and hair follicles.

 ➤ C: Connective tissue. Underneath the skin is the fibrous tissues connecting the skin and scalp

 ➤ A: The aponeurosis layer of dense fibrous tissues

 ➤ L: The loose areolar: a layer of fat, cartilage bone, tissues and major blood vessels; this is the reason why an injury on the scalp would have lots of bleeding. This layer is sometimes referred to as the "danger zone" because infectious agents can spread into the skull.

 ➤ P: The pericardium provides nutrition for the bone with the ability to repair the damage. It can be lifted in surgery to get to the skull.[39]

---

[39] https://en.wikipedia.org/wiki/Scalp

❖ Oily hair: excess oil glands

➢ Shampoo and rinse with organic apple cider: 2 ounces in a 16-ounce glass of filtered water.
➢ "Super Group" Healing Water spray twice a day to refresh hair. Gently brush to take dirt and oil away.

❖ Baldness and Hair Loss

➢ Baldness: Blend cedarwood, lavender, rosemary, and clary sage in equal parts. Massage into scalp and bald spots on your head.
➢ Use this concoction to massage the back of your neck and spine as well. You can use a bath brush to brush it into the spine all the way down to the tailbone.
➢ Oils for Hair Loss: Rosemary, lavender, cedar wood, thyme, ylang-ylang oil, clary sage, cypress, laurel, lemon, roman chamomile, sage, wintergreen.
➢ Add any of these oils to jojoba and grape seed carrier oils and massage into your scalp daily. Mask and condition your hair with natural stuff to fight hair loss: Potatoes + Eggs+ Honey helps hair growth.
➢ Massage hair with cold press virgin olive oil or organic cold pressed coconut oil, wrap hair in a warm towel for 20-30 minutes or overnight for hair loss.
➢ Massage hair with essential oils (7 drops of lavender, tea tree oil in the jojoba oil, wrap and soak hair for 15 minutes.

113

Hair Naturally
Rinse hair with mixture water and apple cider vinegar for pH balance.
Or warm tea water – white tea can help reduce and protect UV damage.

Homemade recipes:
❖ Celery leaves and lemon juice. Apply on the scalp before rinsing can help hair growth and reduce dandruff.
❖ Eating eggs, rosemary tea. Aloe-Vera is good for both hair and skin.
❖ Egg mask, yogurt, and honey masks help hair to grow stronger.

Hormone imbalance and deficiency can:
❖ Cause extreme hair loss.
❖ Menopause phase discomfort.
❖ Stress in pregnancy.
❖ Imbalance in hormones

Knowing your hair condition and choosing the right method to fix it is essential.

➤ Chemicals, like ammonia, and hydrogen peroxide, in hair coloring, will damage your hair by drying up the shafts, killing follicles and even poisoning your brain.

➤ Depending on your hair condition, washing your hair daily-over washing-may not be good for your hair. If your hair is thinning and does not grow back, wash every other day instead.

➤ Drying with a high heat for extended periods and over brushing is not good for your hair.

➤ Cure dry ends and split ends with hair masks, biotin, and folic acid.[40]

---

[40] http://www.homeremediescare.com/10-natural-home-remedies-to-get-rid-of-hair-split-ends/

- Take plant (natural not petroleum) vitamins: C, A and E and Keratin to help hair grow.
- Superfoods: black sesame seeds, organic turmeric, and papaya leaves help overall health.
- Release stress by deep breathing with the diaphragm–see 30-second belly breathing for good health.

❖ Natural Treatment for Hair

- Use organic, natural products for your hair.
- Do not over brush and comb over rough tangled hair as it will cause breakage.
- Do not brush hair when wet. Comb with large tooth comb instead.
- Use rounded tip hair brushes to prevent scratching the scalp.
- Massage your scalp or comb your hair while watching TV.
- Nutrition is essential for hair growth. Asians eat black sesame seeds to grow shiny long and healthy hair to reverse gray hair to black hair.
- Gray hair is a battle for many years, even with good nutrition; besides coloring it's hard to change hair color back. NSP Chlorophyll ES, Liquid has Copper, could help to retain black color for hair. [41]
- Take natural herbs such as horsetail for hair and needs of Silica.
- Dandruff is dry skin on the scalp. It can be itchy and embarrassing. Using lemon juice to rinse and

---

[41] http://theyouthdoctor.com/?sn=1483-5

a celery leaf mask can help. Taking supplements can also help (coconut oil–fatty amino acid).

- ➤ Cactus plant, garlic, onion and cinnamon sticks– I've never tried these, but many say they are helpful.
- ➤ Some have suggested adding birth control pills to the shampoo–LOL
- ➤ Infections, like ringworm fungus, should be treated as soon as possible. Check with your doctor.
- ➤ Hormones are the chemical messengers needed for complex body activities in cells and organs. [42] They are transported to cells via the bloodstream. Endocrine system glands, like the thyroid, adrenal and pituitary glands, generate different hormones and coordinate with the nervous system to regulate growth, energy, sexual functions, and homeostasis [43].

❖ Healthy Hair Growth

Hair needs vitamin A and C, and Keratin to grow. Essential fatty acids and zinc help hair growth.

Hair needs other things such as iron, calcium, folic acid, and biotin. Iron deficiency is the lack of healthy red blood cells. Red blood cells are made in bone marrow and carry oxygen to the cells.

Folic acid is essential vitamin B. It helps DNA and the body to make new cells.

---

[42] https://draxe.com/10-ways-balance-hormones-naturally/
[43] http://www.dictionary.com/browse/homeostasis

Dull color and damaged hair can be caused by over exposure to sun rays, coloring, bleaching and perm.

For damaged hair because of illnesses, find out what your body constitution type is and take supplements and organic foods that help you to rebalance your health.

Other super foods are organic Turmeric, Organic Black Sesame Seeds, Broccoli Sprouts, and Shiitake mushrooms. Beware of the quality of the super foods. [44]

❖ Sacred geometry for hair

Rebecca, my hairdresser friend, is learning Sacred Geometry for hair, and she says that making Sacred Geometry patterns for hair will help too.

Once again, I have been using Apple Cider Vinegar to rinse my hair after washing for a couple of months now. Hair is soft and subtle with that remedy. The hair also starts growing at my bald spots now. Check out the status report at my website for the progress.

Herbal vinegar hair rinses help with oily hair: Put 2 cups of filtered water in a glass jar. Add rosemary, lavender and let it sit in the sun for a couple of days. Then remove the herb, add 2 ounces of apple cider vinegar, and use it as shampoo.

---

[44] http://www.foodsafetynews.com/2016/08/six-brands-of-turmeric-added-to-recall-for-excessive-lead/

Both men and women can benefit from brushing hair techniques

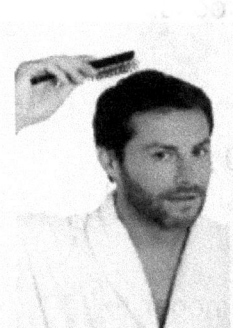
Dreamtime -ID 22630336

❖ **Be gentle with your hair and scalp**

Brushing the hair twice a day for a few minutes can help keep your hair and scalp healthy.

Spray with herbals to refresh and clean hair.

❖ In Asia, Buffalo Horn combs with wide teeth are very popular, although they can be a little sharp and can damage your scalp. These combs are beautifully hand carved and used mostly as ornaments and special occasion gifts.

❖ If using a natural or synthetic brush and comb, choose brush with rounded tips, to prevent damage to the scalp.

❖ Your head has many acupressure points, so brushing and massaging the scalp can relax your head, stimulate your brain, and help hair growth.

❖ Combing with Buffalo Horn Comb or comb

Combing: Divide your hair into two even halves. Use the comb to press down and move ½ inch from the forehead all the way to the hairline of your nape. Comb each line on the right and left sides of the head four times.

Combing with buffalo horn does not create static electricity like a plastic comb does. It also helps to treat follicles and spread natural oils to your hair.

It does give a sense of refreshment to my scalp when I use the comb. Some of the comb's teeth are sharp, so beware and do not comb too hard if that is the case.

❖ Massage head and hair and brushing

Massage the scalp after applying essential oils to help your scalp and thinning hair.

> ➢ Put your thumbs on the back of your head, fingers up front. Gently massage from front to back, and back to front. Apply essential oils on your fingers if desired.
> ➢ Brush hair front to back, follow the 9 imagery lines, then bend forward and brush back to front along these lines. Brush each side of head 9 times, front and back. Take a few minutes in the morning and evening to do so.
> ➢ Spray with the herbal spray to refresh hair before and after brushing.

❖ Brush your back using the bath brush if desired.

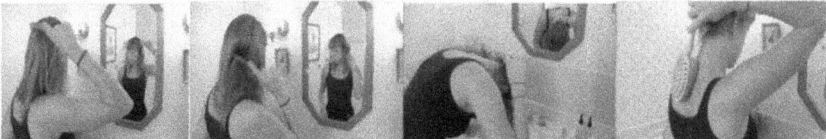

Chapter 7: Hair & Scalp—Summary Box

1. Journal your hair type: Oily hair due to excess oil glands, dry hair with split ends or brittle hair with itching scalp, normal healthy hair.

2. For dry scalp and hair: (muscle test) zinc, flax seed, hair mask with olive oil, eggs, coconut oil.

3. Doc D's advice: Take **natural silica** to improve your hair texture and thickness. HSN-W (hair, skin, and nails) is a good product with natural silica in horsetail herb.

4. The Ionic Mineral with Acai, 3 bottle beautiful hair: Find more information on *FunHappyStore.com*

5. Daily gently brush hair, massage scalp, and acupressure to stimulate hair growth.

6. Chlorine in swimming pools can damage your skin and hair badly. Wear a swimming cap, wet your hair before going to swim, and rinse your hair with an organic rinse after swimming.

7. To prevent split ends, rub them with a mixture of drops of lavender, rosemary jojoba in organic coconut oil.

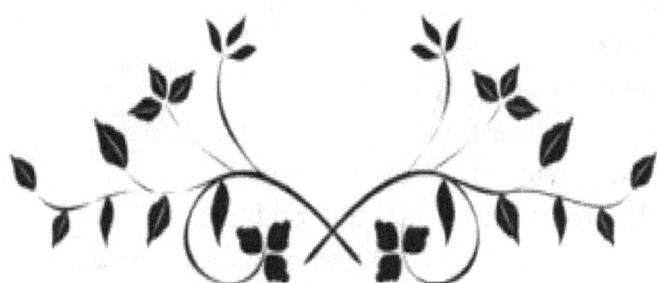

This page intentionally left blank.

Chapter 8—Mouth & Teeth & Gum & Tongue

Teeth and Gum and Tongue Test

- Are your teeth white or black or yellowish? ➜ you might need calcium and vitamin D and other supplements.
- Do you have mercury fillings?
- Put your tongue behind your teeth and feel them. Do they feel solid and strong or do they feel thin and fragile?
- Are they loose or do they hurt when you chew food?
- Are they sensitive to hot or cold liquids?
- Are your teeth clean without calcium buildup?

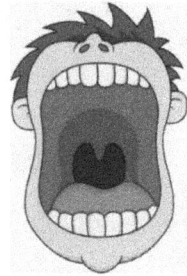

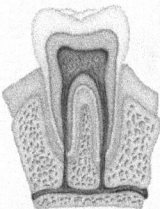

bigstock-Dental-
Anatomy-4803498.jpg

- When you brush, do your gums bleed easily?
- Are your gums pink and firm?
- Are your gums receding? Do they feel sore?
- Do you have bad breath?
- Is there solidity in the gum?
- Is your tongue pink and clean?
- Lift your tongue up, look on the sides and under and notice any unusual signs.

Mouth

❖ *Part of the throat chakra (communication system ➔ the voice)*
❖ *Part of the digestive system.*
❖ *Part of the relationship system kissing, loving, caring.*
❖ *Part of the expression system.*

Amazing Tongue

❖ *10,000 taste buds.*
❖ *The only organ capable of sending taste to the brain.*
❖ *Saliva keeps the tongue moist to detect taste.*
❖ *Women have shorter tongue than men. Women smile more often than men!*
❖ *There are 600+ bacteria on the tongue. Saliva has millions of these, causing bad breath if tongue is not cleaned.*
❖ *Flexible, playful and sensible, the tongue is needed for eating, talking and kissing.* ☺

• Feel the roof of your mouth by curling your tongue up and notice the sensations. This point connects to connect to your pituitary and your pineal gland.

The mouth consists of two lips to cover what is inside the mouth and to protect the throat against foreign objects. The lips outside are soft, movable, and serve as an opening for food intake and part of the process of speech. They are a sensory system, kissing, and showing emotions. Pouting lips and smiling are all parts of the lips functions.

Mouth and throat are made of soft tissue. These connect to the lungs and the stomach and your nose. Fumes and air go right up to your brain when you breathe. So beware of your environment and the air around you to keep yourself healthy.

Having good oral hygiene is having the good habit of good health. It adds to your total well-being; as the

123

condition of tissues and structures in the mouth affect the physical body.

Brush your teeth and clean your tongue in the morning and evening. I even brush after meals when possible.

Don't forget to check up with your dentist every 6 months!

Your mouth, teeth, and the tongue are part of your digestive system. They help chew foods, making small enough pieces to swallow. They also affect your ability to speak and have relationships with others.

Yellow and rotten teeth are not pleasant to be around, let alone kissable!!! Keeping your teeth healthy is important.

❖ Care for the mouth, throat, lips:

➤ It is very painful when your lips are dry and chapped. If it is not because of the weather like winter, then it could be a sign of vitamin B deficiency. To help moisten the lips, use the balm to moisten them.
➤ Others lip diseases are cold sores and canker sores; these usually take a couple of weeks to heal.
➤ Throat itch and irritations: Pay attention to them. Gargling with Himalayan salt and water can help in healing them quickly.
Spraying with Herbal Super-Group Healing Water daily can help.
➤ Dry mouth is another disease of the mouth. it is saliva drying out, making it difficult for the mouth to function in swallowing and chewing. There are many reasons for dry mouth: stress, aging, nervousness, medication, etc.

Saliva is necessary for the food digestive system. Chew your food well. Massage your face and mouth. Put the tongue on top of the roof of the mouth while breathing deep helps produce saliva.

"There are millions of bacteria in one drop of saliva." [45] Saliva can contaminate water in a few hours. Don't drink left over water and don't reuse thin bottle plastic water, especially if it is left in a hot temperature in the car.

Spray with Super Group Healing Water twice daily in the mouth and nose or when needed to clean mucus, virus and harmful chemicals.

❖ Teeth and Gums

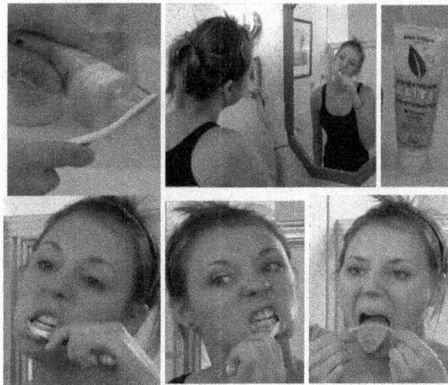

➢ Our teeth are our chewing mechanism of our digestive system. It is a sign of the beauty of our face: smile, pink lips, and white teeth. So we don't want to lose our teeth because when you lose your teeth, your face features are going to look different, right?

➢ Take care of your teeth, meaning brushing, flossing, and brushing your gums too. Brush your gums every day. I like to use an electric toothbrush; it is more efficient in my opinion. Remember your mouth is an opening to the

---

[45] http://www.brighthub.com/science/genetics/articles/45935.aspx

outside environment and for food intake; there is lots of stuff around, so make sure you use organic mouthwash to help your mouth in fighting infections and bacteria.

➤ Brush and floss to clean between teeth.
➤ Brush teeth: 2 minutes–Electric Toothbrush and Organic toothpaste. Brush upper, lower, left, right, and surfaces.

➤ A tongue Cleaner is good for cleaning bacterial build-up, food debris, fungi, and dead cells. It can help bad breath and improve your taste buds.

Do not swallow the toothpaste; rinse it out to help your stomach.

❖ Brush Teeth and Gums Techniques

1) Brush your teeth with the brush angle at 45 degrees.
2) Use circular strokes with the brush in a gentle scrubbing motion. Let the electronic toothbrush stay on the teeth surface about 10-20 seconds each.
3) Do the same thing on top of the teeth and inside of the teeth.
4) Brush the gums in front and both sides up and below teeth.
5) Brush the inside part of the gums behind the teeth.
6) Let the bristles of toothbrush go between the teeth to take out plaque.
7) *Some people even brush the tongue; I use tongue cleaner instead.*
8) Choose a toothbrush with soft, end-rounded bristles. Change your toothbrush every few months as the bristles are broken and can become sharp and damage the gums.
9) The gums are a placeholder for your teeth. You need to brush them to keep them strong and healthy.
10) Rinse with an organic herbal mixture.

11) Gums are sensitive. Help them prevent infections and bacteria.

12) Food and plaque can get stuck between teeth. You'll need dental floss to remove them. The toothpick is used a lot in Asia.

** There is "baby floss" nowadays on the market. These are inexpensive and convenient. You may want to use them instead.

Toothpaste: Recently there are many reports of the harmful effect of artificial fluoride. It is very harmful and toxic.

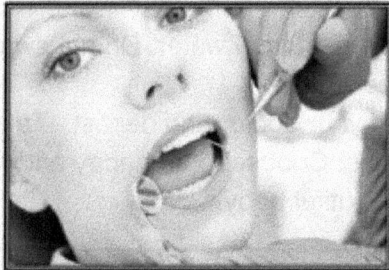

A pregnant woman's dental health can affect her unborn child.

http://wow-content-club.com/

Pregnant Women & Dental Health

❖ Beware of hormone changes; it may have an effect on the gums.

❖ To prevent pregnancy gingivitis, floss and clean between teeth well, twice daily and between meals. Use an electric toothbrush and organic toothpaste – Artificial fluoride may not be good for you and baby.

❖ Brush upper, lower, left, and right surfaces. Brush gums: upper, lower, inside, and outside.

❖ Choose a tongue cleaner to clean and remove the bacterial build-up, food debris, fungi, and dead cells. This can also help eliminate bad breath and improve your taste buds.

❖ Rinse well with herbal water. Do not swallow the toothpaste.

❖ Check with your doctor and dentist. Take multivitamins. Choose to be happy and have a healthy, beautiful baby!

**A NOTE ABOUT ORGANIC TOOTHPASTE AND MOUTHWASH: To be on the safe side, I buy toothpaste without fluoride and make organic mouthwash at home. You can find many companies selling dental products without the chemical fluoride.

Children and pregnant women should not use fluoride toothpaste
content.time.com/time/specials/packages/article

www.youtube.com/watch?v=nbjsvA8eTNQ
Fluoride destroy collagen synthesis and affecting
prezi.com/yshqtlarfj0a/trial/

❖ How to Prevent Decay through Nutrition

When the mouth is acidic, tooth decay can occur. The acid levels of your mouth increase if you eat a lot of starchy or sugary foods. By avoiding foods like this, you can prevent decay.

Detox the mercury fillings with herbal products and Healing H.A.P.P.Y Bubbles Systems ™

Take multi-vitamins for teeth: calcium, iron, vitamin B complex, and vitamin C. Muscle test or use the Magic Scanner to find what NSP herbal products your body needs.

Check with your dentist when needed for cavities, gum disorders. and yearly clean-up.

Avoid foods like candies, cookies, cake, pie, sugar gum, soda pop, and other sugary liquids. It does not mean you eliminate them forever. Eat them on special occasions only, and enjoy!

Processed sugar is not good for you anyway; instead, eat fresh fruits, vegetable, and sprouts.

Use raw honey for your glucose needs! Raw honey has many benefits for health and can even heal some illnesses.[46]

Once or twice a week, brush with mixture of coral calcium or sea calcium, some drops of enzyme water, and a few drops of essential oils

Make sure you floss after eating and, if possible, brush your teeth.

---

[46] https://draxe.com/the-many-health-benefits-of-raw-honey/

Black Teeth Beauty: Before modern society invented the toothbrush, the tradition of blackening the teeth was practiced in many ethnic groups of East Asia, For example, the Yunnan: Hmong, Lahu, Yao people.

- Viet Nam: Vietnamese, Dao Tien, Lu, Black Hmong, Nung people.
- Laos: Hani, Katu, Phu Noi people.
- Thailand: Akha, Lisu people.
- Pacific Islands: the Philippines, Marianna Islands, Palau, Yap.
- Japan: Ohaguro tradition - " Yellow teeth are a real turn off, but black teeth are a major turn on, for the ancient Japanese peoɩ le, at least. Ohaguro simply means to blacken the teeth."

    "Ohaguro, the Japanese teeth-blackening custom.
    https://heritageofjapan.wordpress.com/2012/08/29/the-ohaguro-the-japanese-teeth

Chapter 8: Mouth, Teeth, Gum, and Tongue— Summary Box

1. **The mouth** is the beauty and emotional and voice and expression of a person – Keep it healthy!
   a. Chapped lips can be caused by dehydration, sun damage, weather condition. Put a natural lip balm in your dresser to use it at night.
   b. Other lips diseases may come from malnutrition, chronic illnesses and/or virus, and bacteria. Check with your medical doctor.

2. **Tongue and teeth and gums:**
   a. Detox to get rid of harmful chemicals.
   b. Use a good toothbrush. Change it often to prevent scratching of the gums.
   c. An electric toothbrush is best, especially for children and the elderly.
   d. Floss or toothpick after eating with handy baby floss. Brush gums twice daily also. It is vital if you want to keep your teeth!
   e. Clean your tongue with tongue cleaner twice daily to get rid of bacteria, fungus, and viruses in saliva.
   f. Check calcium, manganese, zinc, vitamin A, B, and C levels

3. Spray your mouth, nose, and throat with Super-Group Healing Water to prevent bacteria, viruses, radiations, and chemicals from doing harm to your mouth and health. It also keeps your breath fresh.

4. Enjoy your pearly, beautiful, white teeth and smile a lot!

Chapter 9—Acupressure Points

Acupressure points, called "tsubo" in Japanese, are the end of nerve points that conduct bioelectrical impulses in the human body.

Ancient acupressure techniques trigger points to release tension and increase the circulation of blood, heightening the body's vital life energy to aid wellness. It also used for a preventive measure to keep the Chi of the body vigor and fit.

A trained acupuncturist does acupuncture with needles. Acupressure uses gentle but firm finger pressure. You can do yourself anywhere, anytime.

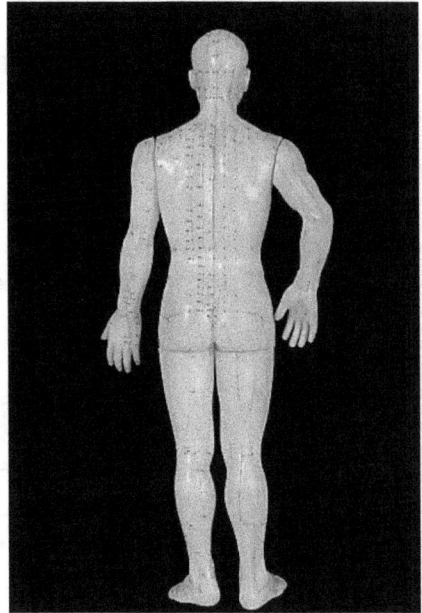

Acu-body-Bigstock_1122387

Do twice daily in bed before going to sleep and before getting up, if desired.

Applying pressure to acupressure points on the face can bring "Chi" energy to it by releasing blockage in the area. After using cream and serum, practice pressing these points daily.

Oriental tradition tells us this is like a facelift and may support a young, vibrant face for years to come. Stop immediately if you experience extreme pain. Pregnant women should not use acupressure. Check with your medical doctor.

Use prolonged and steady finger pressure directly on the point. Usually, the point is a tiny indentation at the edge of a bone. Each point feels different; some points feel tense, while others can be sore or ache when pressure is applied.

Find the balance between pleasant and firm pressure pain hurt and releasing hurt (similar to the "good, relaxing hurt" you feel with a massage).

Experiment with different points to help you choose the ones you like for your daily routine. Practice others in your free time for fun. There are hundreds of acupressure points on the human body.

Disclaimer: This is for general information and practicing home-use techniques only. This is not the official teaching of the Acupressure Institution and is not intended to treat any medical condition.

Pressure points
(Do the following for a maximum 5-10 minutes twice daily)

Using One Finger, Four Fingers, or Your Knuckle:

- ❖ Press and apply pressure gently, hold for 2-3 seconds.
- ❖ Stop if you feel excruciating pain.
- ❖ Do not push on the eyes.
- ❖ Don't forget to breathe: With your tongue on the roof of the mouth, breathe in deeply through the nose for 5-10 counts, then out through the mouth for 5-10 counts.

Do Acupressure Daily on Your Face:

- ❖ Eyes and Eyebrows
- ❖ Cheeks
- ❖ Nose
- ❖ Mouth
- ❖ Jaw
- ❖ Ears
- ❖ Back of Head and Spine
- ❖ Nape, Top of Back and Spine

**Pregnant women:
Do NOT practice Acupressure!**

Ｆace & Ｈair Ｈead Ｈairline & Ａcu-temple Ｌift

Pressure Points (Do for only 5 to 10-minute maximum)

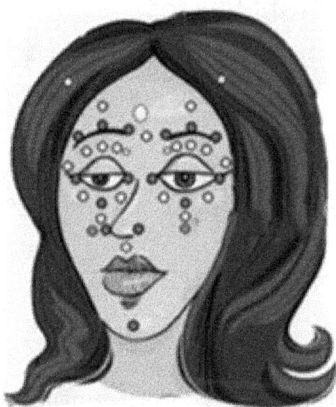

The face has quite a few beneficial points:

Third eye: connecting with the pituitary point, it is between the two eyebrows. Pressing and massaging it will relieve head congestion and headaches.

Gently press on the forehead to relieve headaches and stress.

Hair and Head Acupressure, Massage or EFT [47]

Massage hair and head to prevent headaches and pressure to the skull and brain. **It is a good exercise for the brain!**

Imagine there are nine lines on the head from hairline to nape: a middle line and four lines on each side of it.

[47] http://eft.mercola.com/

- ❖ Use fingers or knuckles to press, massage or tap and move your fingers down the central line from hairline of the forehead to the back of the neck and continue to neck bone and spine.
- ❖ Press or massage or comb the points on each line on the side of the head.
- ❖ Do this three times for each line.

❖ Hairline and Forehead

- ❖ Press across the hairline to the temple and down next to the ears with your fingers three times. Each tiny crevice is an acupressure point: it helps to prevent hair loss.
- ❖ Press upward along the hairline and back 3 times.
- ❖ Press on the forehead from middle toward the temple, and then back.

❖ Eyes points and under the eyes are beauty spots.

- ❖ Pressing, tapping or massaging them will prevent wrinkles and give you glowing healthy skin. Frankincense oil is excellent to rid of wrinkles.
- ❖ Do these along with a face massage and exercise for a few minutes each day.

❖ Use fingers or knuckles to press, massage or tap; along the eyebrows, the corner of the eyes and gently below the eyes.

❖ Do three or four times for each spot.

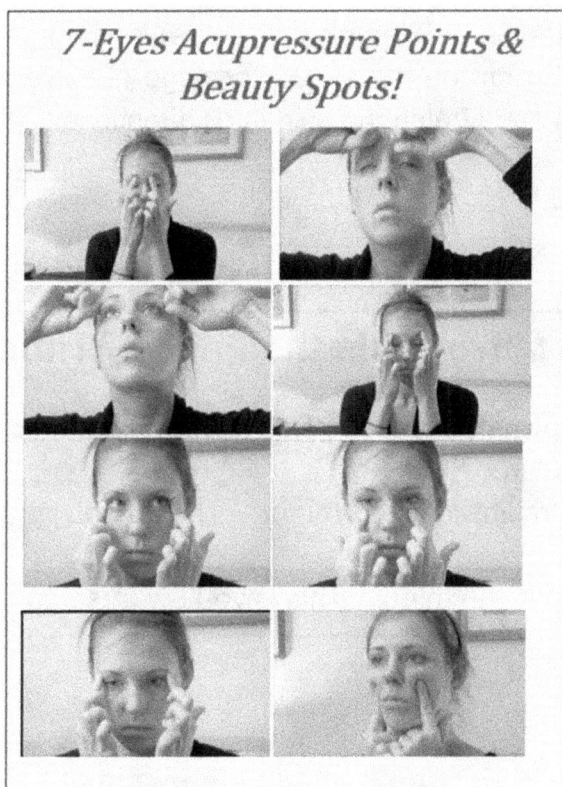

7-Eyes Acupressure Points & Beauty Spots!

❖ Acu-temple lift

❖ Press firmly on crow's feet, near the outer corners of eyes. Palms and fingers on sides of the head.
❖ Till head down slightly while pulling and pressing on temple up with heels.
❖ Smile, mouth slightly open. Breathe in deeply, breathe out slowly, six times.
❖ Place fingertips on temples. There is a large circular groove between the top and outer ridge of the ear. Press gently, pull and stretch the skin in all directions.

The Mirror tells the Face of Time!

➢ Look down in a mirror: This is you 5 years from now in the future.
➢ Look straight into the mirror: This is you at present time.
➢ Look up in the mirror: This is you 5 years ago.

Acupressure for the Nose, Philtrum, Mouth, Chin & Collarbone.

Nose points help improve breathing, relieve nasal blocks, cold and flu.

❖ Press lightly on the nose's bridge, from top to bottom three times.
❖ Use fingers or knuckles press on the side of nose down and around points next to nostrils.
❖ Do three times on each point.

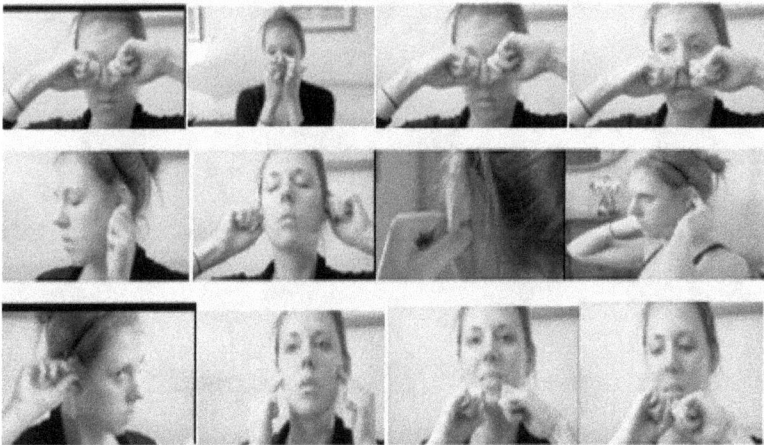

Philtrum, Mouth, Chin, Jaws and Collarbone's massage, EFT tap or acupressure will help the gums, double chin, and even constipation ☺

❖ Press on the philtrum (GV 26) with fingertips, massage clockwise help with nose bleed, fainting, recover consciousness.
❖ Press around the mouth.
❖ Use your index finger and thumb put pressure on middle of chin (double chin and constipation) ☺
❖ Use both hands index finger and thumb, press and move outward from chin to base of ears.
❖ Use the right hand to press on left collar bone, front and back.
❖ Use the left hand to press on right collar bone.
❖ Press on the middle of your chest also helps the lymphatic system.

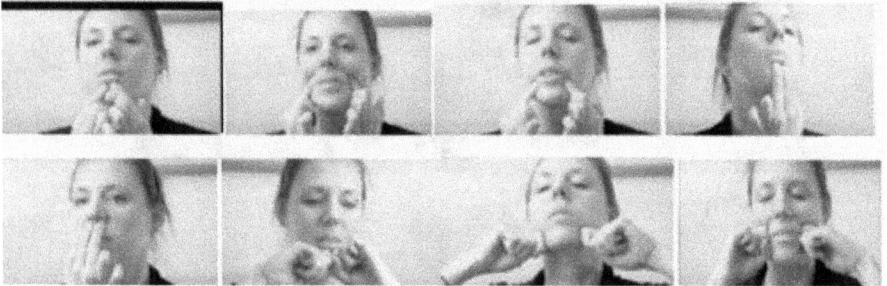

Ears have about 150 points in each one. Press and massage around them to help many organs in your body. The outer ear is the spine area and relieves back pain. Earlobe massage brings energy to you and will wake you up!! ☺

❖ Ears are vital for hearing and to maintain balance..
❖ Use thumb and index finger and press each ear on the outer auricle from top to earlobe.
❖ Press fingers and massage each earlobe for a few seconds.
❖ Use knuckle press inside of ears. Use both thumbs, press behind ears, all the way down to middle of jaw to help the lymphatic system
❖ Massage or press deep behind the ears, where the connection of ears and brain is. If there are sensitive spots, circle them gently.
❖ Especially for headaches, ear pressure, tinnitus and TMJ (Temporomandibular Joint Disorder – hinge of jaw not working properly):
  • Hold two fingers on both ears, down on 2 points (ST19, TW 21 – Triple Warmer), located in the middle of the front opening of each ear. Move the jaw gently for 30 seconds. Repeat three times.
  • TW 17 (right below the earlobes to treat ear itches, facial spasm, and jaw pain. [48]

---

[48] http://www.modernreflexology.com/acupressure-points-for-jaw-pain-and-tmj/

Lymphatic system massage
(http://www.drdavidwilliams.com/lymphatic-system-drainage-exercises/)

➢ To help drainage of waste out of the body
➢ Lymph travels one way to the heart
➢ Massage behind ears, under arms, nape, neck gently down toward the heart.

Clearing Clogged or Ear Infection with Frankincense Essential Oil.

➢ Spray NSP Silver Shield liquid on Q-tip, put a drop of Frankincense essential oil on it.
➢ Gently clean inside the ears
➢ Put a drop of Frankincense oil on a plastic ear wax cleaner, clean out the clogged ear wax
➢ Use a clean Q-tip, spray NSP silver shield liquid, put a drop of Frankincense oil on it. Clean the inside of your nose, gently and deeply clean the nasolacrimal duct.
➢ In 15-20 minutes, you might hear popping or tension. You might even smell the scent in your nose or throat. You might feel irritations in the ears.
➢ That means it is working! Great, now you can hear again! Test with the headphone, compare sounds.
➢ Leave it overnight. You will be amazing to find more of the wax inside the ears. Do the cleaning again, twice a day for 7 days.

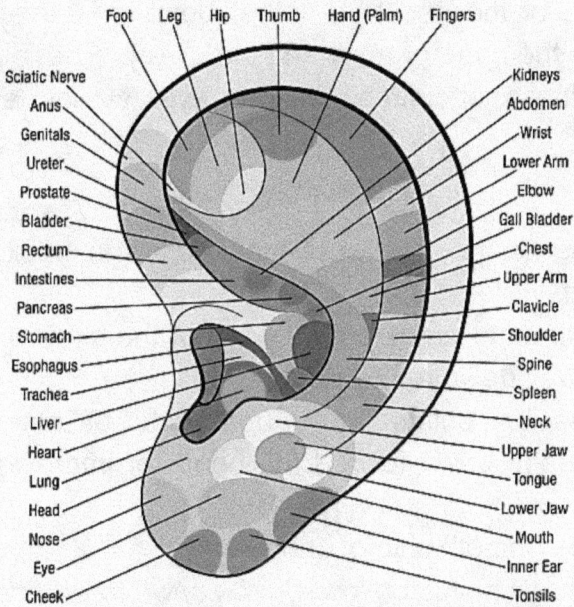

Ear Reflexology Chart

bigstock-Ear-reflexology-chart-descript-68880139.jpg

Back of Head, Nape, & Shoulders

The back of head, nape, shoulders, and along the back of the spine has many pressure points such as Shoulder Well (almost at the base of the neck). Another point is Heaven pillar (half way across the base of neck and shoulder). These points could reduce stiffness, shoulder pressure, eyes strains, even asthma and spasm.

- ❖ Press on points under the hairline in back across the head.
- ❖ Continue to press on the base of the skull in the back all the way down to the spine.
- ❖ Press on points along both side of nape; can also massage down toward the heart for improving lymphatic system.
- ❖ Press on both side of shoulders,
- ❖ Press on points on lower back down to tail end.

Massage the Gate of Consciousness points, releases endorphins, natural feel-good substances. These are neurochemicals produced in the brain's hypothalamus and pituitary gland.

144

Gate of Consciousness, Wind Pond, GB20, One Point Healing

The hollow below the base of the skull, on both sides of the neck, between the two vertical neck muscles, is acupressure point GB20.

GB20's other names are Gate of Consciousness, Wind Pond, or One Point Healing. These are potent points in acupressure; they relieve pain by releasing endorphins.

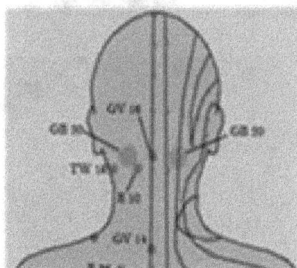

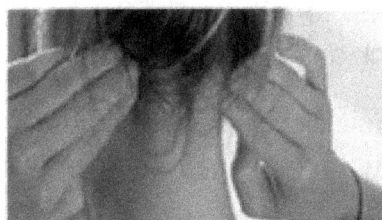

Palming Eyes, Ears, Neck, Collarbone or Any part of the body

Palming brings the warmth energy to an area to relax it. It is especially good for the eyes, and releases pressure when wearing glasses and for working a long time on the computer. It can also improve eyesight.

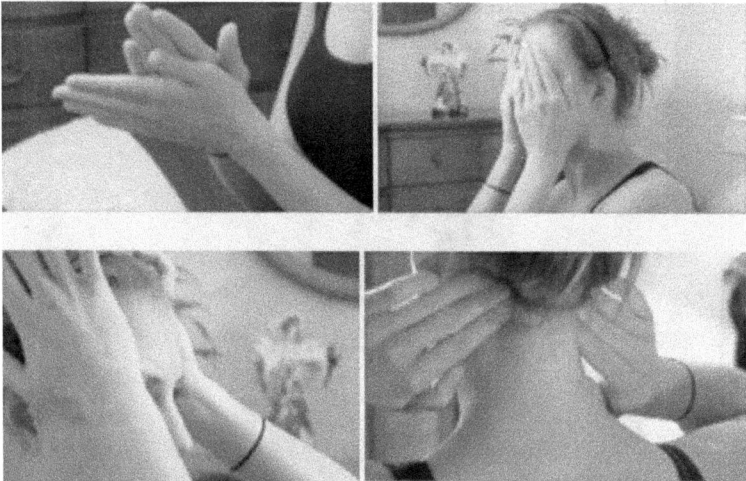

Palming can be done to any part of the body to bring "Chi" and energy balance back and to release pain.

Rub hands together clockwise 36 times or until feeling the warmth – Use a couple drops of your favorite essential oil.

- ❖ For eyes, put both palms on the eyes and open them wide, then close tightly, relax, breathe, smile, and hold for 10-30 seconds. Repeat three or four times. This can be done at bedtime to induce sleep.
- ❖ Apply to other areas: cheeks, temples, back of head, heart, stomach, etc.
- ❖ Breathe deeply, relax, enjoy!

Can be done anywhere, anytime to refresh and rejuvenate:

These palming and acupressure techniques can release pressure and physical discomforts such as headaches, and many other pains.

They are easy to do. Use them anytime during the day to relax the body, mind, and even spirit.

Breathe deeply and don't forget to smile. Applying a few drops of organic oils on your fingers when pressing on the scalp, the back of the neck and the shoulders can help to relax them even more.

Hand Feet Massage & Pressure Points

Hand and foot acupressure and massage are important. It is like giving your inner organs a treat!

There are 28 points on the hand: [49]

> ➤ If you're using a professional service, drink a glass of water, and eat one hour before and after the session.
> ➤ Warm your hands before massage by putting a drop of essential oil in both palms. Warm them up again by rubbing circularly 9 times.
> ➤ Spray herbal water or put cream on fingers to moisten them, then on top of the hands and inside the palms.
> ➤ Move in small circular motions on painful spots.
> ➤ Hand Valley Point (between thumb and index finger): Relieves stress, toothache, neck pain, and inflammation.
> ➤ The base of thumb point: can relieve coughing.
> ➤ Massage each finger then knit both hands together for the spots between the fingers.

Massage and press on the whole hand, wrist, fingers together

❖ Pull each finger outward to relax the joints.
❖ Tap or EFT and stretch to complete the session.

---

[49] http://www.newhealthadvisor.com/Acupressure-Points-in-Hand.html

Hands Massage & Pressure Points

❖ Massage fingers and wrists.
❖ Massage and relax your large intestine by pressing or tapping the point between thumb and index finger.
❖ Hold the whole hand including the thumb, squeeze gently. This will massage the opposite side of the brain: Left hand for right brain. Right hand for left brain.
❖ The right brain is your creative part.
❖ The left brain is the logical part of you.

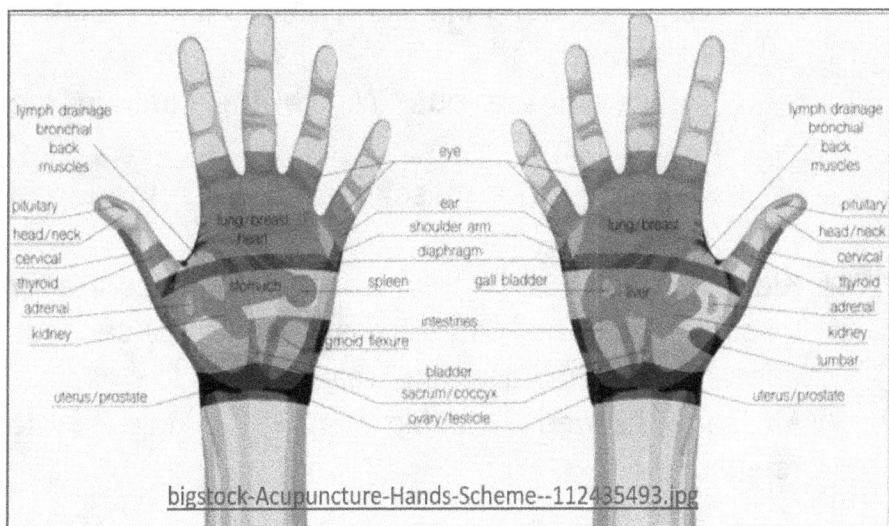

lymph drainage
bronchial
back
muscles
pituitary
head/neck
cervical
thyroid
adrenal
kidney
uterus/prostate

eye
ear
shoulder arm
diaphragm
spleen   gall bladder
intestines
sigmoid flexure
bladder
sacrum/coccyx
ovary/testicle

lung/breast
heart
stomach

lung/breast
liver

lymph drainage
bronchial
back
muscles
pituitary
head/neck
cervical
thyroid
adrenal
kidney
lumbar
uterus/prostate

bigstock-Acupuncture-Hands-Scheme--112435493.jpg

Feet Acupressure Points: Feet maintain our balance and connection with the Earth. The 8th chakra is below the feet. You carry it with you all the times. The feet are the most acidic parts of the body; everything goes there.

- ➤ If you are using a professional service, drink one glass of water. Eat and drink one hour before and after the session.
- ➤ Warm hands with 1 or 2 drops of essential oils.
- ➤ Spray with herbal water, put on some cream.
- ➤ Breathe, relax, start with left foot and ankle then the right foot.
  - o Press with 2 fingers: Start with tops of each toe: the 5 meridian points connect with the brain.
  - o Press on toenails, knead hand between the toes.
  - o Squeeze along the side of the foot 3 or 4 times for few seconds.
  - o Pull each toe out. Wiggle the toes in the sockets.
  - o Tap or EFT or massage and press the top of the foot.
- ➤ Kidney 6 and B 62 on both sides of the ankle are for insomnia. Hold both and press them for 30 seconds a few times in bed. Breathe, relax and go to sleep.
- ➤ Massage between the big toe and middle toe to release anger.

- ➤ There are many other points in feet that you can massage. We use a general approach to massage the
- ➤ KD1 (Kidney 1) in the middle of the foot also helps release hypertension.

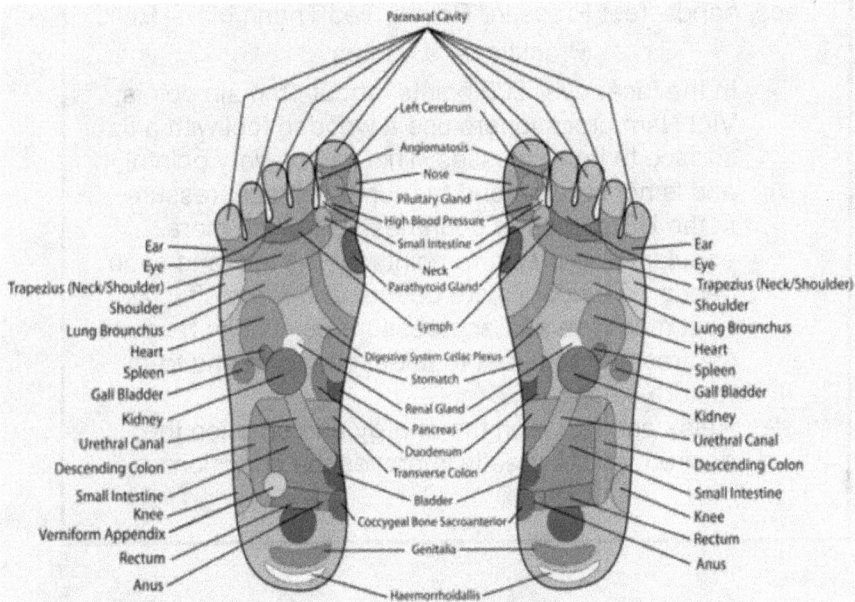

bigstock-Traditional-alternative-heal--65691994.jpg

Face, hands, feet Pressure Points: Ted Thanh Mai – Reiki Practitioner's quotes:

➢ In the face, over 500 points, about 15 main points, Viet Nam practitioners use a wooden tool with a flat surface to heal illnesses. This can be very painful, and is not recommend for home self-acupressure.
➢ In the US and other countries, it is much more popular to do pressure points for the feet and even hands.   The points are deeper and more effective.
➢ Foot massage and acupressure points can be done for tired and hurt feet to release tension and to restore balance.
➢ Relax and focus on the energy and envision the desired results greatly improves the conditions.

Chapter 9: Acupressure Points— Summary

1. World Health Organization recognizes about 400 acupressure points on the 12 meridians in Chinese medicine. There are many more points.
2. Take a few minutes each day before bedtime and in the morning to massage the main points. It will really help you.
3. Spray herbal water or use essential oils and cream for enjoyable and a softer touch to the skin.
4. If there are arthritis spots on the knuckles, use Dissolve cream of Uncle Al.
5. Cracking noises in the joint joints are sign of mineral deficiency. Take Ionic Mineral with Acai from NSP.
6. Make angel wings flying with hands to enjoy the feelings or wellness.
7. Put your hands together to massage the points between fingers.
8. Acu-press between your toes for different benefits: between toe 3-4 to improve eyesight.
9. Sing or listen to healing sounds when

Chapter 10—Workbook

Summary

❖ **Eternal Youth Secrets**

1. *Understanding what you want and why you want it. Ask for help and allow help from Earth and Divinity Teams*
   For example: If you want to be healthy, to enjoy life, look good, to be productive, able to work and to help your loved ones, you are not alone in the universe. As a matter of fact, you can't do everything alone. There is help always available for you. You just need to ask and allow.

2. *Choose Good Health and Happiness. Accept the help.*
   You can have it all, health, wealth, beauty. Synergy the energies, know the values you provide for yourself and the world. Reflect your inner beauty inside out, outside in.

3. *Do, take actions:* Learn, master the skills you need to manifest the life you want. Become a valuable team player.

4. *Expect total health, envision your Happy Life.* Clear blockages, traumas, release fears, heal hurts with energy healing. Continue to grow and expand with Grace to be in Timeless existence. Tap in the Eternal Youth of your Being.

Truth + Goodness + Beauty + Grace = Eternal Youth

❖ Simple Skincare Methods

1. Your expression of health and happiness reflect in your skin. Moreover, skin is part of the imperative structure of human life. Taking good care of our physical being is our job, using all available tools, selectively, from modern technologies to muscle testing to ancient secrets; whatever is best for your skin, body health and beauty is a wise thing to do. ☺

2. It is simple to take care of your skin: Protect, Prevent, and Maintain.
   a. **Protect** against malnutrition, negative energy, harmful chemicals and harsh the environment. Beware of toxins in your water and food products and packages. *For example: don't reuse thin bottle plastic of water.*
   b. **Prevent** with proper nutrition, happy thoughts, detoxification; usage of good products (barrier creams and oils), healthy skincare habits.
   c. **Maintain and Express** your beauty with awareness. Apply strong hygiene habits, DNA repair (yes, you can change your DNA energetically and help telomeres regrow) and loving resonances (learn to release constraint energies by sending back to the senders – no need to know who it is, even to yourself – 10,000 times of blessings)

3. Detoxify with homemade, natural organic fruits and organic essential oils. Utilize Healing H.A.P.P.Y. Bubbles Systems.

4. Exfoliate face, do face mask and hair mask every 2 weeks.

5. Stretch, Exercise and Practice Tibetan Fountain of Youth.[50] Jump on a trampoline 15 minutes a day will increase your lifespan 5-10 years.

---

[50] https://en.wikipedia.org/wiki/Five_Tibetan_Rites

❖ Cleaning and Caring and Nurturing

1. Read UPC code and labels when choosing products to use.
2. Clean face twice daily with beneficial products.
3. Brush face, skin to take out dirt, bacteria daily.
4. Brush and floss your teeth well, twice a day; and after meals.
5. Massage (preferably with a clean face (no make-up) after brushing or in bed before sleep. Using upward motions on the face. (the best machine I found so far is Nu Skin spa system).
6. Exercise your face anywhere, anytime (perhaps privately). ☺
7. Acupressure anywhere, anytime combined with palming and hands/feet massage to take the stress out of daily functioning.
8. There are many pressure points on head, face, neck, collarbones and chest.

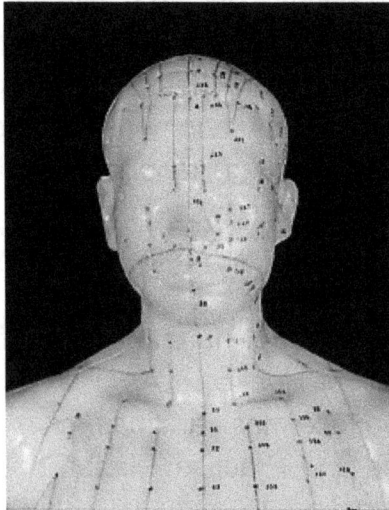

Acuhead Bigstock_1122492

Massaging, Exercising, Acupressure for both men and women (do some, do all, do a little, do a lot, do every day – Take notes, journal, notice the difference)

1. *Main purposes: Relax, remove blockages, improve energy flow, balance and restore harmony in skin, muscles and bones.*
2. Start with head, brush, press or scratch on scalp from front to back (9 lines: middle of head, 4 each side) – Breathe deep.
3. Massage both ears, on top, inside, around, behind ears. Pull earlobes down a few times. Pull ears up to help with the winkles along the mouth (nasolabial folds).
4. Make face, stick tongue out, stretch. Puffing cheeks, have a good laugh.
5. Open eyes wide, blink. Rotate eyes slowly clockwise and counter clockwise 3 times each.
6. Stretch your neck, moving your chin and jaws, open mouth wide, sing like an opera singer. Have fun.
7. Press the acupressure points, along the hair line, eyebrows, nose, cheeks, back of neck, edge of eyes gently.
8. Massage & press neck, back of neck, shoulders, stretch, pull to bring back into sockets.
9. Massage and press collarbones, chest, lungs, ribs, underarms, stomach, bones on sexual organ, tail bones.
10. Massage and press hands, arms, elbows, feet, knees, legs.

❖ Air: The most important element

1. Essential for life.
2. Earthlings will die within 3-5 minutes without air.
3. Many types of breathing and thinking: learn to breathe deep to benefit the capillaries. (tiny blood vessels in the body).
4. Clean air with essential oils and Healing H.A.P.P.Y. Bubbles.

❖ Sounds: Vibrations of communication

1. Open secrets, communication, connection and alter lives.
2. A human can't live without sounds.
3. Silence is a sound; space is a vibration. Silence and space are needed for vibrations to transmit.
4. Use sounds to nurture your skin, your body: self-talk.

❖ Food: joy and love of life

1. Evolve into a host of art and gourmet cooking.
2. Without nutritious and proper foods, you can become ill.
3. There is a difference between malnutrition and under nutrition
4. Eat for health, joy, and grace.

❖ Water: abundance of energy

1. Everything needs water. It is a life source and a vibration.
2. Without water, things become dry, dehydrated, and dead.
3. Drink clean water ½ of your weight daily, in 4 Oz portion. Beware of contamination by saliva.
4. Learn to transform ordinary water into blessed water for your body, car, house, bank accounts. ☺

❖ Don't forget LOVE

1. Love is essential for life. Everything needs love.
2. Without love, life has no meaning. It is empty and limited.
3. Love is a skill: self-love, love, being loved, receiving love.
4. Love with respect, be open to love and be loved for no reason.

Nutrition

1. *Did you laugh today? Laughing 15 times a day is the best nutrition for everything. Smile counts too. Pamper yourself with beauty & goodness!*
2. Provide the body daily needs 90 nutrients from outside sources: 60 minerals and trace minerals, 14-16 vitamins, 3 EFA (Essential Fatty Acids)
3. Use herbal, natural products so your body can Assimilate, Circulate the nutrients and Eliminate the waste. (Doc D. ACE principles)
4. Air, Water, Food, Sounds and Love: Skin needs protein, fat, glucose, vitamins, minerals and trace minerals. Learn to breathe deeply to benefit your capillaries.

Don't forget Love!

5. Meditate. Clear traumas, Programming Brain beliefs and Mind and Body and Spirit in harmony and balance.
6. Use the "Magic Scanner" to find essential herbal nutrition for your body's needs. For more information, please visit:
www.FunHappyStore.com
7. Use Bio-Tracker to measure 8 areas of your physical markers.

Detoxifications

Homemade Remedies

You can make simple drinks at home from essential oils and fruits. Do gentle daily detox by drinking water with 1 drop of oil. Detox with specific products once every 3 months in 15- or 30-day lengths.

Note: Please use filtered water and good quality oils. There are many good companies with essential oils out there. However, we use Nature's Sunshine products as we are most familiar with them.

Below are 4 recipes for cleansing the digestive, kidney and heart, from Natural Body Detox. (n.d.). Retrieved from http://natural-detox-diets.blogspot.com/ [51]

Body Detoxifier - Lemon Zest Black Pepper Cleanser

This recipe is good to clean the colon and the entire digestive system. It is good for the colon and entire digestive system.

- 8 Ounces of Water
- 2 Teaspoons of lemon zest
- ½ Teaspoon of black pepper or one teaspoon of fresh lemon juice to the mix.

Combine the water and the other ingredients and drink it down. After you are finished drinking the solution, drink two 8 ounce glasses of water. This will help flush the solution into your

---

[51] Natural Body Detox. (n.d.). Retrieved from http://natural-detox-diets.blogspot.com/

160

system. For best results, use fresh ground black pepper and fresh lemon zest from a fresh organic lemon.

Body Detoxifier - Italian body detoxifier

- 8 Ounces of filtered Water
- 1 Teaspoon of flax seed oil
- 1 Teaspoon of Basil
- 1 Teaspoon of Oregano
- ½ Teaspoon of Garlic

Combine all of the ingredients with the water and drink it. After drinking, wait five minutes for the solution to settle and then drink two more glasses of water. This acts as a detoxifier for the entire body and is good for both the digestive system as well as the circulatory system.

For best results, use fresh herbs and garlic.

Alternate use - You can substitute Rosemary for Basil.

Body Detoxifier - Berry Detox

- 6 Ounces of Water
- 2 Ounces of Pure Acai Berry Juice
- ½ Cup Blueberries
- 4 Fresh Strawberries

Use the blender to mix all the ingredients together. Drink them and follow the solution with an 8-ounce glass of purified water. This is a detoxifier that is loaded with antioxidants and purifiers.

Body Detoxifier - Kidney Cleansing [52]

- 8 Ounces of Water
- ½ Cup pure cranberry juice
- ¼ Cup Pure Acai juice
- 3 Teaspoons orange juice

Mix the ingredients together and add them to the water. Drink it down and then drink two more 8-ounce glasses of water. This will help clean out your urinary tract and clear up urinary tract infections.

For best results - Use only pure ingredients and 100 percent pure orange juice

Body Detoxifier - Vitamin Cleanser [53]

- 1 Cup Green Tea - Hot
- 1 Capsule of Vitamin D
- 1 Capsule of Vitamin A
- 1 Capsule of Vitamin K
- ½ Teaspoon of Cinnamon

Grind up the capsules in a mortar and then add them to the hot tea so that they dissolve. Then add the cinnamon to the mix. Drink it down. This will add vitamins and nutrients to your body that you may be lacking. It is good for eliminating stress, depression and also healthy for the heart.

---

[52] Natural Body Detox. (n.d.). Retrieved from http://natural-detox-diets.blogspot.com/
[53] Natural Body Detox. (n.d.). Retrieved from http://natural-detox-diets.blogspot.com/

Aromatherapy Remedies

Drinking solutions is one of the best ways to detoxify the body. Using essential oils can also work to detoxify your body.

- Essential oils should not be used directly on the skin, with the exception of Rose and Lavender, as they can cause a reaction.
- For children and elderly, open the cap, and wave the bottle below their nose to smell.
- Clear the air in hotel by open the cap and wave the bottle to the whole room and all corners.
- Spray hotel bed, bathroom with herbal water.
- For me, I love to inhale directly by using two drops of the balm. Use your finger to move the oil around, and then cup both hands to your nose to inhale the scent.
- Use pure essential oils or extracts only from reputable sources. Synthetic oils will not give you the same results.
- These recipes are all safe to use topically as massage oils. Inhale oils allow for detoxification through the lungs.
- Use the oil diffuser to clean the air in house and car. Nature's Sunshine has a cute small portable diffuser that you can put in your purse.
- Use Super-Group Healing water to clean public toilets, and airplane or bus seats. It is very useful, and works very well.
- Take bath with a few drops of your favorite oils. It is so relaxing and calming, as the water and oil go through skin to your bloodstream taking out the toxins.

Aromatherapy Body Detoxification - Lavender and Rose

This is one of the easiest of all of the aromatherapy detoxification recipes, although rose oil is very expensive. It combines two of the safest essential oils that will not only relax you, but cleanse your body of its impurities.

* ½ Cup Lavender Oil
* ¼ Cup Rose Oil

Mix well together and then massage onto your feet, neck, and chest area. The essential oils will be absorbed into your skin and then into your blood stream. This is a good recipe for those who are tense and want to relax while detoxifying their body at the same time.

Aromatherapy Body Detoxification- Frankincense

Frankincense has been used as a healing potent for thousands of years. It is expensive but it works extremely well.

This can be used as a way to get rid of body toxins, help circulatory system, cuts, skin wrinkles and many other uses.

* 1 Cup Carrier Oil (such as canola oil)
* 1 Teaspoon of pure Frankincense

Mix the oils together well. You should put them in a dark bottle with a cork lid for the best results. Once they are mixed together, you can then use them as a massage oil. Rub the soles of your feet with this mixture as well as the chest area. This will do wonders for your circulatory system and the scent is pleasant. If you have a partner, see if they will massage your back. Have fun!

Aromatherapy Body Detoxification - Tea Tree Oil and Lemon

Both Tree Tea Oil and Lemon Oil are useful when it comes to helping the digestive system. If you want to lose weight as well as clear out your digestive system so that it works well, you can make this mix at home and use it as a massage oil or in an infuser:

- 1 Cup Carrier Oil (such as canola oil)
- ½ Teaspoon of Tea Tree Oil
- ½ Teaspoon of Pure lemon oil (not lemon juice)

Mix the oils together in a brown bottle and shake. Use them in the same manner as you use the other aromatherapy massage oils.

Put Tea Tree Oils on insect bites or small cuts to help the itches.

Aromatherapy Body Detoxification - Almond

This is one of the aromatherapy treatments that you can use from extracts that are readily available in the health food store. You should still use a carrier oil when you are using extracts.

- 1 Cup Carrier oil (such as canola oil)
- 1 Teaspoon of pure Almond Extract
- 1 Teaspoon of pure Vanilla Extract

Combine all of the products and shake well in the bottle. You can then apply on the skin. The scent is very nice and you can also burn the oils on their own in the infuser. This is a body detoxification that will work to bolster the immune system and clear out any toxins.

Awesome Yogurt Honey Egg Hair & Face Mask!

My favorite hair and face mask. Very simple and so easy to do. Enjoy!

 * ½ cup organic yogurt
 * 1 tablespoon raw honey or organic honey
 * 1 raw organic egg
 * 1 or 2 drops of organic essential oil. (Frankincense or Lavender)

Mix all the ingredients together well, let sit for 5 minutes or put in microwave for 10-15 seconds.

Apply on scalp, hair to tips of hair, wrap in plastic cap, then towel. Rub on face and let it dry naturally. Leave on 20 minutes. Wash hair and face normally.

Notice the hair shaft and the face skin afterward. Beautiful!!!

Nature's Sunshine Essential Oils and Herbal Products [54]

A few samples of Nature's Sunshine products I use and find effective. Besides having great quality products, NSP provides exceptional educational and support for its members.

1. Breathe Deep: cooling, relaxing, clearing.
2. Changes: women's health, changes and PMS
3. Core: balancing, quiet insight, productive.
4. Essential shield: soothing, cooling, bath.
5. Frankincense oil: open cuts, wrinkles, depression, infections.
6. Inspire oil: uplifting, inspiration, motivate, creativity.
7. Lavender: calm, relaxing, skin moistening, sleep inducing.
8. Lemon grass: purity, tone skin, elevate mood, deer repellant.
9. Lemon oil: face skin blemishes, age spots, crisp, clean.
10. Peppermint: work out, indigestion, bad breath, ticks, clarity.
11. Recover oil: muscles soothing, penetrating, warming.
12. Rosemary: hair, scalp, emotional balance, memory.
13. Tea tree oil: insect bites, cuts, skin lotion, hair shampoo.
14. Tei-Fu oil: insect bites, energy, refreshing mind.
15. Silver Shield: clean parasites, infections, molds, cuts.

1. All Cell Detox: clean colon, kidneys, liver, aid digestion.
2. Astragalus: Help regrow telomeres (caps on DNA) for youth.
3. Chlorophyll ES, Liquid (16 fl. oz.): clean blood, deodorize body, retain hair color.
4. Collartrim: Facelift in a herbal bottle – 8 capsules a day for 30 days ➔ 10 years younger!
5. Curcumin BP: anti-inflammation, powerful anti-oxidant
6. DHEA-M and DHEA-F: "Youth renewal herbs: Anti-aging, energy.
7. Heavy Metal Detox: support liver, bind and remove heavy chemical, absorb heavy metal ions.
8. Ionic Mineral with Acai ➔ Beautiful hair, 3 bottles in 4 weeks!
9. NSP Enviro-Detox: remove pollutants and toxin.
10. Tiao He Cleanse (15 day): cleanse intestinal, digestive, circulatory systems.
11. Skin Detox: pull toxins from skin, support structural system.
12. Yeast and Fungus Detox: maintain healthy yeast and microflora.
13. Enzyme Spray: bio-degradable, no cleaning agents, plant-derived enzyme, safely breakdown stains and odors.

Why GMO-free? Why read labels and UPC codes?   Why muscle testing? Why clear traumas?   Why Nature's Sunshine? Pure Herbs, Doc D. and Uncle Al Private Labels?

There are quite a few people that ask me these questions; these are my answers below:

❖ While there is evidence that household chemicals can be harmful to your health; nobody knows for sure if certain products and processes are harmful for people's health or not.

❖ For our group in NJ, we are taking the safe and natural ways to handle our health by using selected tools and resources.

❖ There are many good companies out there; we, however, do not recommend anything that we don't personally use and where we have seen positive results.

❖ It is like when you are sending your children to school or college. In choosing the educational institution, you consider many factors: reputation, quality, safety, distance and cost among several other things, right?
If there are potential dangers to your child, such as influences from untrustworthy, unsafe groups or organizations that could be harmful to your children and damage their life forever, would you still want to send your children there?

❖ Living a life in sickness, dependency on others, being a burden to a loved one and society is not a fun thing to do.

❖ In the US, we spend millions, billions of dollars to fight illnesses every year.[55]

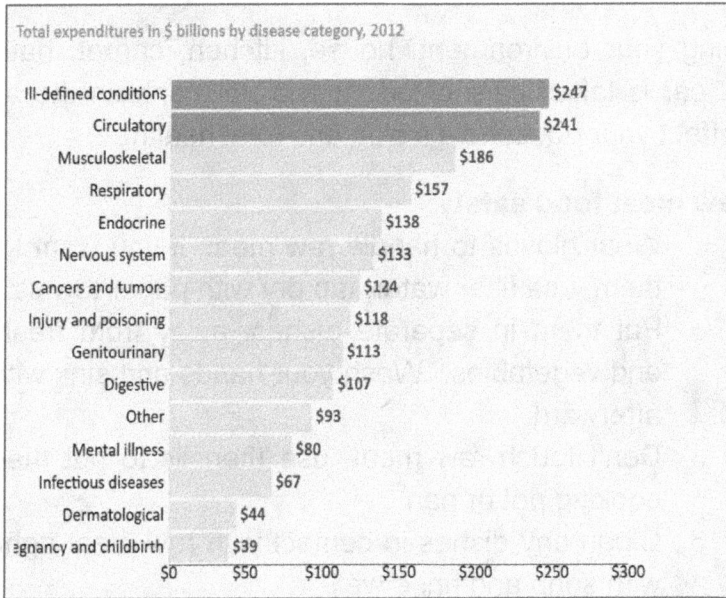

Total expenditures in $ billions by disease category, 2012

Ill-defined conditions	$247
Circulatory	$241
Musculoskeletal	$186
Respiratory	$157
Endocrine	$138
Nervous system	$133
Cancers and tumors	$124
Injury and poisoning	$118
Genitourinary	$113
Digestive	$107
Other	$93
Mental illness	$80
Infectious diseases	$67
Dermatological	$44
Pregnancy and childbirth	$39

❖ Taking a few minutes, a day to ensure that you are in good health and continue to be in good health; is it worth the time and effort to you?

❖ In your hands, you are holding one of most powerful, mysterious, innovative and fun systems, created and never seen before. The choice is yours. We hope you come and join us in the adventure to explore Health, Beauty and Wellness of your own.

❖ Please visit: www.FunHappyStore.com for more details on the "Eternal Youth Methods" and the "Money Goodness with the Magic Scanner" online training. Thank you!

---

[55]   http://kff.org/slideshow/how-much-does-the-u-s-spend-to-treat-different-diseases/

Cleaning Essentials

Cleaning your environment: house, kitchen, carpet, bathroom, foods, car is taken care of odors and pollutants in the air, that may affect your household's skin and total health.

❖ **Raw meat food safety:**
  o Wear gloves to handle raw meat; if you want to wash them, use filter water, tap dry with paper towels.
  o Put them in separate dishes, away from fresh fruits and vegetables. Wash your hands and sink with soap afterward.
  o Don't touch raw meat, use utensils to put them in a cooking pot or pan.
  o Clean any dishes in contact with raw meat right away with soap and rinse well.
  o Spray with herbal water then dry right way.

❖ **Fresh vegetables and fruits:**
  o Put 3 tablespoons organic apple cider in water.
  o Add 1 teaspoon of organic or Himalayan salt.
  o Wash fruits gently in the water.
  o Cut and clean the vegetables and let them soak in this water for a few minutes.
  o Shake them dry in the plastic colander, and let dry naturally, or tap dry with clean paper towels before putting in storage.

❖ **Clean portable drinking cups, car:**
  o Clean them daily. Saliva has bacteria and can contaminate water easily. Dry and spray with herbal water.
  o Open windows. Spray your car with herbal water.

- ❖ **Clean kitchen, dryer, washer, dishwasher:**
  - o Clean kitchen, pots and pans, dishes right after usage to prevent bacteria and contamination build-up.
  - o Clean dryer filter after use right away so the dust does not fly in the air or get on the carpet and become stains.
  - o Run washer with NSP Enzymes Spray and essential oils to rid of odors, mildews and molds.

- ❖ **Clean house, beds, bathroom, carpet:**
  - o Set up a day and time 1-2 hours for cleaning weekly.
  - o Open garage doors, windows, turn on fans in kitchen, bathroom, let the fresh air comes in.
  - o Clean trash can with herbal spray.
  - o Clean bathroom floor and toilet weekly. Put a couple of peppermint oil on a cotton ball and leave behind toilet seat to refresh the air.
  - o Clean bathtub after taking shower or bath right after shower or bath to deter molds, bacteria contamination.
  - o Dust and sweep the floor before vacuum.
  - o Spray herbal water (peppermint, tea tree oil, citrus oil) along the edge of doors and windows to repel spiders and ants. (Spray this herbal mixture before cleaning the garage with open doors to get the spiders out first)

- ❖ **For babies, sensitive skin and elderlies:**
  - o Use NSP Enzymes Spray with one or two drops of Frankincense oil. Spray their clothes, beds, pillows.
  - o Refresh pillows, blankets, bed covers by putting them in the dryer for 10 minutes with herbal spray.
  - o Clean private parts after shower, bath and using the bathroom with herbal water.

Daily Refresh with Healing H·A·P·P·Y Bubbles Systems. ™

Do it every morning, or anytime, anywhere:
- ❖ Breathe in Heaven and Earth
- ❖ Connect to Healing H.A.P.P.Y Bubbles
- ❖ Ask Divine Team to connect HHB with the subject(s)–or yourself.
- ❖ Use the command: Clean, clear, heal.
- ❖ Next command: Download, install, circulate fresh, beneficial air.

For more details of using Healing H.A.P.P.Y Bubbles Systems, please visit: www.FunHAPPYstore.com;

Power Breathing for Napping and Deep Sleeping

1. Put tongue of roof of mouth. Feel the sensation. Breathe in slowly through the nose, pull Heaven energy down all the way down through your feet to center of the Earth.
2. Feel Earth energy, ask her permission to love You, and ask her permission to love Her. Feel the Love, pull up the energy from the center through your feet all the way through the head to meet Heaven.
3. Pull this energy down to your heart, and let it flow, circulate all over you. Note the sight, sound, sense.
4. Give first statement: "Connect to Heaven and Earth". Give second statement: "Activate Healing HAPPY Bubbles" Third statement: "Connect HAPPY Bubbles to me". Download Peace & Calming, deep relaxing, deep restful sleep.
5. *Advanced programming: "When I choose to wake up, I will wake up peaceful, happily, full of energy, feel fresh, and full of vitally.*

6. Continue to breathe in Heaven and Earth and drip into restful sleeping; with wonder dreams.

Chapter 11—Common Sense Doc D. Assimilation, Circulation, and Elimination (ACE)

ACE of Doc D. – Our Super Group's Leader

Assimilation: The function of taking in nutrition such as foods, water, and dietary products to convert them into nutrients that your body can use. When there are too many synthetic and harmful chemicals inside the body, assimilation is not effective and could be more harmful—i.e., Leaky Gut Syndrome.

Circulation: The body function that occurs after digestion to circulate the nutrients to various parts of the body at the cellular level to benefit all cells.

Elimination: The important function of removing waste from the body.

Doc D. has many talents and gifts. The most amazing one to me is *muscle testing*. He can test to find exactly what people need in herbs and natural products and recommend the proper products for them. He is like a living dictionary of herbs, an encyclopedia of natural medicine. Just ask him a question and he can explain it in full detail for a few hours! LOL.

Please remember: If you don't provide enough nutrition for your body; it will start eating itself! It does this so you can live. Prolonged malnutrition will result in death. Pains, discomforts, and illnesses are the body's signals to tell you it needs food, supplements, air and water or a combination of all these.

ACE (**A**ssimilation, **C**irculation, and **E**limination) is crucial for your health. Learn it and use it and your body will thank you. It is the only body you have, and if you don't take care of it, how do you expect it to work for you?

Doc D. says: The 13 body systems, including blood circulation to the capillaries, are all important for health and wellness.

1- NERVOUS SYSTEM: Thoughts, sensations, emotions signal responses, actions: muscles co-ordination

2- ENDOCRINE (GLANDULAR) SYSTEM: Monitors body, secrets hormones and regulate chemical, hormone, growth and body functions

3-THE HEPATIC SYSTEM: The body's central filter, removing waste and contaminants from the circulatory and digestive systems.

4- URINARY SYSTEM: Works to Filter and remove nitrogenous waste our of blood. Regulate electrolytes, maintaining fluid and pH balance.

5- CIRCULATORY SYSTEM: Provides the entire body with life-giving oxygen and other nutrients while removing cellular waste. Support immune system.

6- RESPIRATORY SYSTEM: Oxygen and carbon dioxide exchange, moisten & heat air.

7- DIGESTIVE SYSTEM: Breakdown foods to nurture body, sustain life and provide energy

8- REPRODUCTIVE SYSTEM: Sexual organs for offspring production, production of hormones

9-STRUCTURAL SYSTEM: Protect inner organs, give strength and structure. Produce red blood cells.

10-INTEGUMENTARY SYSTEM: Skin, hair, nails, largest sensory organ outsider, protect the whole body, vitamin D syntheses, regulates fluid and blood loss.

11- IMMUNE SYSTEM: Network of many systems to protect and defend the body, Fight diseases.

12- LYMPHATIC SYSTEM: Transport lymph (liquid with white cells) to help fighting infections, picks up fluids leaked from the capillaries. Control growth, balance and energy level.

13- MUSCULAR SYSTEM: Muscles create movement, maintain posture, generate heat and blood circulation.

14- SPACETIME: Invisible mathematic fourth dimension continuum; where all events happened at the same time.

Common Sense Stuff

Doc D. and Super Group Tools and Principles

As a rule, we—Doc D. and the Super Group in NJ—only recommend the products we use and that have proven to be effective.

Doc D. has many tools. The most fascinating and newest one is the "Magic Scanner! No more guessing! This wonder scientific tool fits in the palm of your hand! In 2 minutes, it reports 5-10 herbal nutrition your body needs!

We are using it in our Money Goodness projects; to raise 10K-100K for non-profit organizations.

Doc D. is a muscle-testing (Applied Kinesiology AK) expert. He identified the needs of my brain and recommended Blessed Thistle Brain Treatment and Mesoglycan. They helped to heal my brain physically. I then cleared my brain of traumas in tragedies with Theta Healing. Without Muscle Testing, I probably would still be walking in the darkness, never seeing the light.

The In.Form Super Group in NJ is composed of several practitioners in natural medicine. Doc D. has been practicing the longest: 40 years. In total, the group has over 180 years of experience!

Doc D. has several other tools; they are all fascinating! See the following descriptions.

Quantum Life Infinity: measures and balances the vibrations in your body for better health. Really cool!

Compass: Doc D. takes your hand and reads the herbs your body lacks in great detail.

Derma Grid: Doc D. takes a picture of the back of your hand and submits it to the server. It comes back with a detailed list of minerals and trace minerals that you need.

Muscle Testing is very easy to do, especially when you use your fingers. You bring them everywhere with you, right? In a few minutes you can learn this life skill and use it forever.

You can use muscle testing to test for foods, water, editable products to find if they are good for you. Even when I want to eat candies or cakes, I test to see if they are good for me; if no, I test to see if my body can handle it, and how much. LOL!!!

Muscle Testing Techniques

Muscle Testing could be the best and only way to communicate with your subconscious and unconscious mind to reprogram your beliefs and change beliefs that cause suffering to happy, honorable, and successful beliefs.

There are 3 levels of consciousness.

The first level is the **active conscious**; this is the level of consciousness you are in when you are awake, eating, or driving. The second level is the **subconscious**, similar to a computer operating system, holding whatever you programmed or allowed to take root. It controls 90% if not more of your behaviors and health. The third and vast level of conscious is the **unconscious** – universal, mysterious, unknown, wisdom.

3 Levels of Consciousness

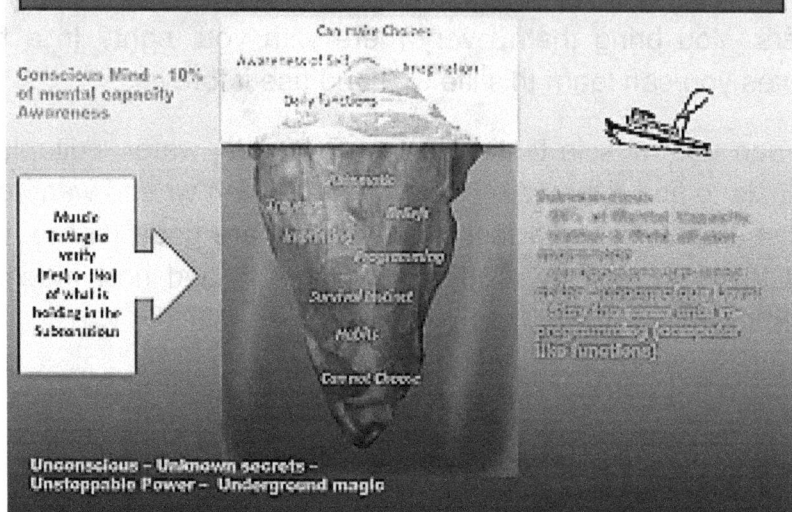

MUSCLE TESTING WITH FINGER CIRCLE METHODS

Make a circle with 2 fingers on the less dominant hand
Ask Yes or No question
If Yes, the circle will not break
If No, the circle will break

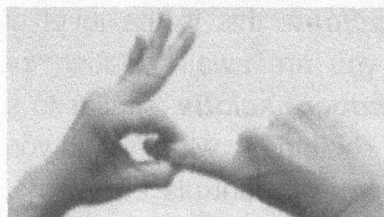

YES answer, circle stays strong, can't break

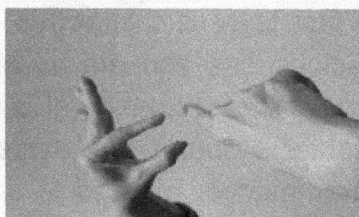

NO answer, circle is weak & breaks open

So let's start

1) **Zip up your energy field** – take your hand and move it from your tailbone all the way over your head, then move your hand sideways.

2) **Form the finger ring, then test Example 1: Test your real name.**

   1- My name is [Your real name] – Muscle Test- answer should be YES, the circle stays strong and will not break

   2- My name is [Someone else's name] – Test: answer should be NO, circle is weak and breaks open.

3) **Do another test: Example 2: Test your real location**

   1- I am at [Your real location: home, state, school, etc.] Muscle Test- answer should be YES, circle stays strong and will not break.

   2- I am at [Somewhere else] – Test: answer should be NO, circle is weak and breaks open.

And you are done! Congratulations!

Now, you can test your food and all kinds of things:

➢ Is this good for me? ➔ if YES, the finger circle will not break.

   ➔ if NO, the finger circle will break open.

➢ If the answer is No, and you still want to eat the food, ask the question: **Can my body handle it?** The answer may be Yes, then you can enjoy the food!!!

You can also test your water and many more things you eat and drink among many other things. Enjoy!

Why Is Removing Toxic Wastes Important?

The skin absorbs everything out there, good and bad, like a sponge. If we don't eliminate the toxins, they will stay inside us and cause malfunctions. Radiation or EMF is one of the hardest things to eliminate. Radiation is everywhere; it is from computers, cell phones, TV, and microwaves.

However, you can clean radiation with Heavy Metal detox of Pure Herbs. NSP also has many detox products. There are other ways to take the radiation out, like taking bath salts and with organic baking soda, to clean the radiation out of the body after an x-ray process.

Removing toxic waste from your body will help maintain good health and skin.

Detoxification will also improve bowel and kidney functions. It is good to ensure that you eliminate toxins daily. Many manufacturers suggest you do colon cleansing two times a year.

Combine these procedures with Healing H.A.P.P.Y Bubbles Systems to clean radiation, harmful chemicals, even parasites, molds from your energy field, etheric, auric fields and the physical body is a complete care solution for your body.

❖ Who Needs Body Detoxification?

Detoxification is a process to remove the toxic elements from the body in order for it to continue functioning or to restore your health.

180

Your body undergoes a lot of wear and tear throughout your day-to-day life. Toxins and free radicals are affecting your organs, your skin, and your overall well-being on the inside and the outside.

> You could be exposed to harsh chemicals through work environment or ingesting harmful ingredients in food.
> Things like cigarettes, acidic foods, caffeine, junk food and soda are all harmful to your health. If you are consuming these things on a consistent basis, you are harming your body on several levels.
> All of these elements working together can cause toxins to build up in your system over time and can cause a whole host of problems including weight gain, memory problems and immune system issues.
> By nature, the body can detox itself. However, when you have a poor diet and a stressful lifestyle your body isn't able to cleanse your system properly.
> If your body is not able to do its job properly, you can take steps to help it so your health can be improved.

❖ Detoxification can:

> Improve your immune system function.
> Eliminate free radicals from your systems.
> Improve your ability to fight off cancer cells.
> Cleanse out congestion and mucous from your body.
> Purify your blood.
> Help you break your addiction to sugar, salt, alcohol and junk foods.

Detoxification is slowly being acknowledged by modern medicine, but there are still skeptics out there. Just about anyone can make use of body detoxification.

Depend on your lifestyle and your health, you can choose how often you want to detox. If you have a lifestyle with habits such as smoking or heavy drinking, you may want to use body detoxification more often. You can detox less often if you are in good health.

Researchers suggest detoxing once every 6 months.

❖ Remove toxins from the Digestive and Intestinal Systems

➢ The liver, pancreas, kidneys, and intestines are organs functioning in the digestive system. The other names are called "Hepatic system" and "Intestinal system."

➢ Foods enter the digestive system from the mouth for chewing, next travelling to the throat and esophagus and then to the stomach.

➢ Then foods go through the processing of the digestive tract. Some foods and drinks make liver, kidneys, and pancreas work harder to process them.

➢ After being processed and convert to energy, the nutrients go to nourish the body. Liquid waste is eliminated by urine; solid waste goes through the large intestine or colon to be discard of as stool. The Intestinal System contains of the colon or "bowel". It function is to rid the body of waste, or stool. It reabsorbs water to be used again.

➤ If there is waste build up on the walls of the colon, it hardens into mucous plaque. This hardened mucus harbors bacteria and parasites and prevents or pollutes water being reabsorbed by the blood upon passing through the colon walls and could cause many problems.

➤ Fiber cleans the colon and exercises it. When fiber is lacking in the diet for a long time the colon becomes weak and constipation can occur. [56]

According to the *Colon News* website, skin diseases such as acne benefit from a colon cleanse. If the colon is not functioning correctly, toxins will make their way to the surface of the skin and erupt through skin pores in the form of blackheads and pimples.

Therefore, a colon cleanse will help to eliminate skin problems such as acne by keeping toxic levels to a minimum and help the colon to function more efficiently.

See
http://livestrong.com/article/32184 3-colon-cleanser-skin-health/#ixzz2AZD5Euhu

---

[56] Herbs That Work – Judy Vedder, C.I, M.H – http://IridologyNYC.com

We recommend using CleanStart to clean your colon.

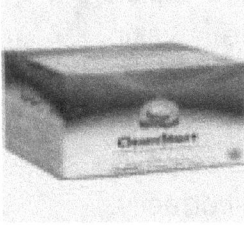

"CleanStart is a two-week program that supports natural waste elimination to provide a sense of improved energy and well-being. It contains powerful nutrients that help cleanse and detoxify the body".[57]

Benefits of using a product such as **CleanStart** from Nature's Sunshine include the following:

❖ Supports the natural, everyday cleansing of toxic wastes.
❖ Works without dangerous side effects.
❖ Improves energy and promotes a feeling of well-being.

Detox Basics (30 day) of NSP – This provides your body with

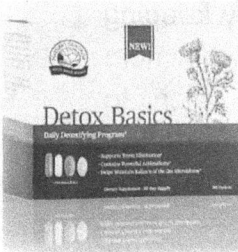

the nutrients it needs to help neutralize, prepare and convert toxins for transport and elimination on a daily basis.

Benefits:

❖ Supports microbiome balance and gut health.

❖ Helps liver, kidneys, bowels in the elimination process.

❖ Contains antioxidants to fight free radicals.

---

[57] http://adf.ly/1ae6wv Clean Start and Research http://adf.ly/1ae89x

❖ Has Vitamin A, N-Acetyl Cysteine (glutathione precursor), Vitamin C, Milk Thistle seed extract, Dandelion root, *Bacillus coagulans* (shelf-stable probiotic), Inositol, Choline bitartrate, Turmeric rhizome and prebiotic fiber (food for probiotics).

❖

❖ Other toxins

The air you breathe can have chemical fumes and toxins going into the circulatory system, and can be harmful to your health. It is impossible to live your life toxin free, even in your own home, if you are not aware of these.

Eventually, you are going to go out in public and pick up germs that are in the air. It is inevitable that you will come into contact with toxins unless you decide to live your life in a plastic bubble.

Smoking is not only affecting your lungs. The smoke is absorbed directly into the bloodstream and can damage other organs as well. Even second-hand smoke can take its toll to your well-being

Then there are chemicals in shampoo and soap. When you take a bath or shower, you can be absorbing toxins into your skin.

❖ Detoxification Benefits and Process

➢ **Lose weight:** Detoxification will get rid of the waste in your body and you will feel much lighter. Your body can process foods and nutrients more efficiently. It is one of the healthiest ways to lose weight. Body detoxification is not a laxative, and you need to follow a certain procedure properly, like the Detox Basics for 30 days.

- **Heal your body:** It could help your body fight diseases, boost your immune system, prevent illnesses and even heal your body faster.
- **Always look for natural ingredients** that your body can easily absorb. Using chemicals harmful for your body will not help the process at all. Green tea is one the popular components when it comes to weight loss through body detoxification.
- **However, please do not drink green tea or coffee on an empty stomach**. There are reports that excess use of green tea could harm your liver. Using herb tea or papaya tea also can help. Cranberry herb without sugar helps clean out the urinary tract.
- **Avoid harmful chemicals:** Artificial sweeteners, pesticides, preservatives, artificial colors in food that your body can't process or even eliminate.
- **To Rid Yourself of Toxins:** is to keep your body free and clean from poisons in foods, water, and in the air you breathe.
- There are many detox kits in the market available for you to choose. Usually, a period of 7 days to 2 weeks or even a month, are required for the body to adapt to the process properly.
- **Colon cleansers** are popular to help cleaning out the waste before it becomes toxic and harmful to your body. The colonic process may be helpful although it is a process and should be done by professionals only.
- **Detoxification** may not be suitable for pregnant women and should be used every 3-6 months only. Please check with your doctor.
- **Drug detox:** using herbal remedies to clean up the drug residues in your body will help addiction to the drug. Combine with meditation and happy healthy thoughts; you could become healthy the way the want it.

- ➤ **Aromatherapy:** Aromatherapy is good for body detoxification on a long term basis. It does not work quickly, but is effective. It is similar to the patches in that it is absorbed into the bloodstream and works to cleanse all parts of the body, including the digestive system. It works well for those who want to have a long term body detoxification experience at home.

- ➤ **Exercise, stretching, massages, and acupressure** are also essential for body detoxification. Cardiovascular exercises will work up a sweat; relaxing exercises, such as yoga, deep breathing, massages to eliminate stress.

- ➤ **Foot therapy:** Feet are the pathway to your body and foot therapy can work well to cleanse your body from impurities. Feet are the most acidic part of your body, and they are in need of tender care often. Check back to Chapter 9 for feet therapy.

❖ Stay Healthy

- ➤ Skin and body detoxification is not difficult and there are many choices from which to choose when it comes to what type of remedies you want to use. You will get into the habit easily and when you see the results, it even gets better and easier with time.
- ➤ Follow the instructions, and don't starve yourself. It is not safe to suddenly stop eating or losing weight too fast.
- ➤ Nature's Sunshine IN.FORM is one of the best ways to lose weight and detox with the support of a coach in a group setting. There might be emotions arising during the process, and having a coach to help you through these periods is valuable and safe.

- ➢ Detox safety in the protection of Healing H.A.P.P.Y Bubbles Systems™! **Visit www.FunHappyStore.com for available groups with date and time.**
- ➢ Also do not forget to clean your environment (car, home, bathroom) with Essential oil diffuser and be selective when using cleaning products for your home.

Essential Vitamins, Minerals, & Trace Minerals for the Skin and Body

Complex organic compounds are vitamins needed in small amounts for the health of the organism; they are life force carriers. The human body can't produce vitamins, so they must be ingested from outside sources.

Vitamins perform hundreds of tasks in the human body and provide the biochemicals the body requires.

Minerals and trace minerals are essential for growth and overall health. Some minerals the body needs average more than 5g and some trace minerals needed average less than .05mg -. 20mg. As each mineral and trace mineral has a different and significant impact on the body, the ability to absorb them in a form beneficial for the body is the primary focus.

13 essential vitamins: vitamin A, vitamin D3, vitamin B-complex, vitamin C, vitamin E, and vitamin K.

Vitamin A (fat soluble): is important for healthy skin, bones, vision, and hair; cell growth and multiplication.

Dr. Joel Wallach suggested there are 90 nutrients; with 60 essential minerals, 16 vitamins, 12 amino acids, and 3 essential fatty acids.
http://nomdforme.com/faq/what-are-the-90-essential-nutrients/

The Eight B-complex Vitamins (water soluble) help the nervous system, reduce stress; improve energy; aid in metabolism; and keep eyes, hair, liver, mouth, and skin healthy.

Thiamin (vitamin B1) protects nerve tissues. Riboflavin (vitamin B2) works as an enzyme to help create energy and inhibit free radicals.

Free radicals are unstable atoms, and molecules with an unpaired electron, that grasps the electron of healthy cells, causing chain reaction damage. Stress, smoking, the toxin in the environment, radiations, gems, etc. can produce free radicals.

Antioxidants are like the heroes. They can stabilize free radicals, the bad guys!

Researchers have shown the important benefits of dietary supplements in vitamins, minerals, and trace minerals. [58]

Vitamin A affects skin, bones, vision, and hair. Deficiency in vitamin A is linked to conjunctivitis (pink eye), night blindness, and softening of the cornea.

Vitamin A is the basis of Retin-A, used to treat acne, balding and wrinkles. It restores and cures the skin. It is essential for managing cell growth and cell multiplication.

Vitamin D3 is necessary for healthy bones and immune system, brain function, muscle strength; it is fat soluble.

Vitamin D3 deficiency is a problem worldwide. It is estimated that 50,000-70,000 people in the United States and 30,000-35,000 people in the United Kingdom die prematurely from cancer each year due to vitamin D insufficiency.

---

[58] http://www.health.harvard.edu/staying-healthy/listing_of_vitamins

Use vitamin D3, or cholecalciferol, instead of the vitamin D2; it is the recommended form of vitamin D. It is the natural form of vitamin D that your body makes from sunlight. Vitamin D3 is crucial for bones and the immune system. [59] It also facilitates the nervous system and normal brain function, preventing blood clotting and blood cell formation, cardiac activity, and optimal muscle strength. It appears to help with the conversion of blood sugar into energy.

Vitamin B-complex: (B1, B2, B3, B5, B6, B7 (Biotin or vitamin H—the "H" is from the German words for hair and skin, *haar* and *haut*[60]), B9, and B12.

The vitamin B family maintains healthy functioning of the nervous system and might reduce the effects of stress on the body. Their job is to convert carbohydrates into glucose, an energy source for the body to produce energy to function, connecting with ATP. The B-complex vitamins are essential for the metabolism of fats and protein. They help to maintain muscle tone in the gastrointestinal tract. They have an important role for the health of the eyes, hair, liver, mouth, and skin.

Deficiency in vitamin B could lead to *anemia* (where the red blood cell count is less than normal). *Beriberi* is a disease caused by a vitamin B1 deficiency, Thiamine, and affects the nervous system[61].

---

[59] http://adf.ly/1ae8Ov - Vitamin D
[60] http://www.medicalnewstoday.com/articles/219718.php - Vitamin 7 or vitamin H
[61] https://en.wikipedia.org/wiki/Beriberi

Niacin (vitamin B3) aids in cell energy production.

Pantothenic acid (vitamin B5) is in every living cell, crucial for healthy digestion and metabolism and growth.

(Pyridoxine) Vitamin B6 is crucial for the normal function of over 60 essential enzymes, as well as nucleic acids, proteins, red blood cells, immune and neurotransmitters of the brain and nervous system.

Biotin (vitamin B7) increases the body's immune system, fights against Candida, yeast.

Folic acid (folate, vitamin B9) aids DNA synthesis.

Cyanocobalamin (vitamin B12) aids red blood cells and growth.

Symptoms are burning feet, burning and dry eyes, constipation, cracked lips and mouth corners, no appetite, skin disorders, tender gums, chronic fatigue.

High enough doses of B-complex vitamins could treat polio, shingles, and hypersensitive children who fail to react to drugs such as Ritalin. In addition, B-complex vitamins have also been used to treat *alcoholic psychosis* (a mental disorder when an individual loses contact with reality), and barbiturate (an illegal drug) overdoses. [62]

Biotin (vitamin B7) contributes to healthy hair and skin and fights against rashes in the nose or mouth. Deficiency in biotin includes symptoms of anorexia, depression, exhaustion, muscle pain, and nausea.

---

[62] http://www.urbandictionary.com/define.php?term=Barbiturates

Vitamin C-bioflavonoid (different from the synthetic, ascorbic acid) is a natural, water-soluble vitamin that must be obtained from dietary sources. It helps form red blood cells, prevents bleeding and easy bruising, and enhances fine bone and tooth formation. It aids in facilitating other essential nutrients in the body. Vitamin C occurs naturally in most fresh fruits and vegetables. Using copper cook ware can destroy the vitamin C content in foods.

Vitamin Bioflavonoid C has shown with clinical research to have the ability to decrease severe colds. It also could prevent cardiovascular diseases, gum disease and help the body to fight the damages against the pollution in the environment, including cigarette smoke, carbon monoxide, toxin, benzene, arsenic, benzene, cadmium, copper, iron, lead, mercury, and certain pesticides.

Topical vitamin C might be very effective in helping skin look younger. Vitamin C serum might help hair grow faster with more luster.

Vitamin C: An Important anti-stress antioxidant and vital nutrient for adrenal functions. Vitamin C is more concentrated in the adrenal cortex (the size of a walnut, which sits on top of both kidneys). The adrenal system helps regulate metabolism, including the response to stress, with cortisol. Aldosterone helps control blood pressure). Large amount of cortisol reduces the function of the immune system.

Vitamin C helps in the manufacturing of collagen, a protein needed to form connective tissue in bones, ligaments, skin, and nails. It helps speed the healing of burns and wounds by stimulating the formation of connective tissue in scars; it also helps speed up the healing of corneal burns.[63]

The scurvy disorder occurs from a prolonged vitamin C deficiency. Initial symptoms include fatigue; spots on the skin, thighs, and legs; and yellow fever, which if prolonged, can be fatal. [64]

Vitamin E (fat soluble)— has a potent anti-oxidative (molecules help preventing cell damages), it can treat chronic and degenerative diseases such as cardiovascular disease and cancer.

Results from the 1996 Cambridge Heart Antioxidant Study (CHAOS) showed that natural vitamin E (400-800 IU daily) reduced the risk of nonfatal heart attacks by 77% in patients with *coronary atherosclerosis* (plaque in the arteries).[65]

Vitamin E: bones, blood, antioxidant. Natural vitamin E has a higher bioavailability (easy for the body to use) than the synthetic one. Researchers at Oregon State University found that the human body excretes synthetic vitamin E three times faster than natural vitamin E. It helps the immune system, skin, eyes, and brain. It keeps moisture in your skin and nails longer, which helps against toxins from the environment.

---

[63] http://theyouthdoctor.com/?sn=1606-3 - Research Vitamin C of Nature's Sunshine
[64] https://en.wikipedia.org/wiki/Scurvy
[65] Vitamin E - Herbal Remedies - Herbal Kingdom. (n.d.). Retrieved from http://www.herbalkingdom.co.uk/herbal-bible/E/e-vitamin.pdf

Magnesium is reputed to be the mineral most people in the United Sates are deficient in. Seven out of ten people have magnesium deficiency.

Calcium deficiency is also one of the top ten mineral deficiencies in the United States.

ACE Facts—If your body can't assimilate and circulate nutrients to nourish your cells and eliminate waste products from your body, it does not matter how expensive the foods and drinks are that you are taking in.

Enzymes-There are about 75,000 in your body. They are catalysts in metabolic functions, and help with the digestion of food, and come from raw foods.

There is some research saying vitamin E could help fight prostate, lung, oral, and stomach cancer. It might also reduce the effect of chemotherapy peripheral neurotoxicity (chemotherapy produces toxin in the body) [66]

Vitamin K2 helps reduce blood clots and heal the skin. In cosmetics, it is used for spider veins. Even though vitamin K2 deficiency in newborns is rare; doctors will give vitamin K2 injections to premature babies or to those whose mothers took seizure medications during pregnancy.

Vitamin K2: research has shown that vitamin K2 has more benefits than previously thought, including brain health. It helps prevent tooth decay and might help to prevent prostate, lung, and liver cancer.

Vitamin K2, with calcium, is needed to build bone. Low vitamin K causes osteoporosis. [67]

---

[66] http://bit.ly/22r0u11 - Research Vitamin E with Selenium
[67] http://umm.edu/health/medical/altmed/supplement/vitamin-k - vitamin K

Major minerals: The body can't make minerals and trace minerals; they have to be ingested (taken in) from foods and dietary supplements.

➢ Calcium: Is a vital mineral needed for overall health; 99% of calcium is stored in bones and teeth; it helps keep your bones strong. Bone marrow builds red blood cells and contributes to brain health. When there is not enough calcium in your body, it takes the calcium it needs from your bones and teeth, which can lead to osteoporosis.

➢ Calcium helps your skin by supporting cell growth in your skin and by keeping it moist. Calcium also promotes hair growth.

Your skin on your face needs a pH balance of 5.5 to protect against UV rays and toxins in the environment. Potassium helps.

pH stands for the power of Hydrogen, the numeric number from 1-14 describe the level of acidity or alkalinity of a solution.

Sodium is an important ingredient in skin care products. It is also an antibacterial agent used in preserving foods.

Using iodine, thyroid creates the two hormones: T3 (triiodothyronine), T4 (thyroxine), and calcitonin are vital for metabolism functions of the cells.

➤ Silica or silicon dioxide is said to be the most important mineral for human health. It is the beauty mineral and has many functions: It removes toxins from in connective tissues, and it also maintains skin appearance. It also aids in the growing of bones, working together with calcium and magnesium; prevents thinning hair; and prevents brittle nails.

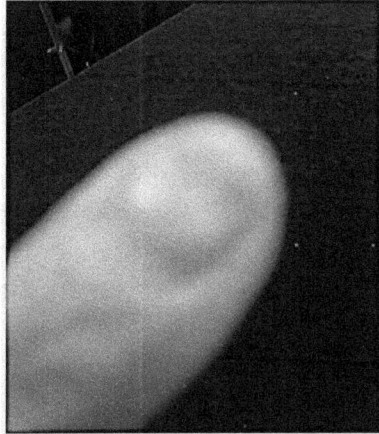
Vicki's finger nail deformed —calcium deficiency

NSP products: HSN-W for Hair, Skin and Nail is one of my favorite. It uses the herb horsetail (has more silicon than any other herbs), dulse, rosemary, sage is a great combination for hair, skin, nail. 68

➤ Chloride: The most important electrolyte nutrient in your blood and body liquids, it is essential in the B vitamin-complex. It helps the fatty production of cell membranes.

➤ Magnesium: Transports calcium into the cells. It is essential in the formation of bone and protein. It hosts enzymes that regulate DNA replication and repair, thus helping to fight against wrinkles.

68 http://theyouthdoctor.com/?sn=945-0

- Phosphorus: Second-most abundant mineral in the body, following calcium. Involved in hundreds of cellular activities in the brain, skeleton, teeth, hormone balance, and is important for your skin health.

- Potassium: Involved in energy metabolism and circulation functions. Necessary for maintaining the pH balance of body fluids. It is an electrolyte (ions essential salt carry electrical charges for muscles contractions) and in every cell in the body. Potassium deficiency causes severe dry skin, called xeroderma. 69

- Sodium: Balances fluids, helps nerve impulses. It is in every cell in the body and plays an important role in maintaining healthy skin, teeth, and hair. Sodium has anti-aging properties. It fights against free radicals to protect the skin. It also reduces mouth odors and cleans and polishes the teeth. 70

- Cooking with natural sodium (salt)—such as celery or Himalayan salt—that the human body can absorb and process is recommended.

- Sulfur: is an abundant mineral in the body. It is a fundamental component of amino acids that are vital for healthy skin, bones, and nails. It helps fight acne, eczema, and psoriasis. It helps unclog pores, controls oily skin and refines the skin's tone and texture[71].

---

[69] http://www.livestrong.com/article/92806-symptoms-potassium-deficiency/
[70] http://www.stylecraze.com/articles/amazing-benefits-of-sodium-for-health-skin-and-hair/
https://www.mariobadescu.com/Sulfur-Acne-Treatment#helpme

Trace Minerals

- Chromium: Stimulates enzymes that are part of glucose metabolism, insulin production, and protein synthesis.

- Copper: Helps the body make red blood and nerve cells. Helps preserve youthful hair color.

- Fluoride – while we need organic fluoride for teeth enamel, synthetic fluoride is poisonous for our bodies.

Free radicals are harmful to cells. They are atoms that have an odd number of electrons. They form naturally in the body when oxygen interacts with molecules. They can grasp and take away an electron from a molecule and thus create a domino effect of free radicals unchecked. It is the pathway for diseases, aging, and even cancer. Antioxidants (molecules to prevent damage of the cells) can safely interact with free radicals and terminate the chain reaction, preventing damages to the vital molecules of the body.

Fat lipids are organic compounds of fat, oils, sterols, and waxes needed by living cells.

- Iodine: Key component for thyroid hormone production, which is crucial for brain development and metabolism. The body can't make iodine; it has to be taken in from food.

- Iron: An active constituent of red blood cells and hemoglobin, which transports oxygen to cells.

- Manganese: Works with calcium to help form connective tissue, promotes blood clotting. It produces sex hormones and boosts sexual energy [72]

- Molybdenum: An essential trace mineral; a cofactor with other enzymes involved in various chemical reactions in the body.

- Selenium: Combined with vitamin E, works as an antioxidant against free radicals.

- Zinc: Helps maintain the sense of smell; triggers enzymes and helps create DNA.

---

[72] http://virilityprotocol.com/essential-minerals-for-virility/

There are over 40 types of skin disorders

Although there are over 40 types of skin disorders, many skin disorders are easily treated with over counter drugs or simple herbal remedies. These could cause embarrassment and discomfort in public.

A few, however, are serious, and could be life-threatening if left untreated.

This book is an effort to raise awareness and awakening to skin health; to prevent disorders by using common sense along with natural herbal products.

Use the magic scanner to find out exactly what nutrients your body need. [73]

The skin disorders could be categorized into 3 groups or by root cause [74].

---

[73] http://www.FunHappyStore.com
[74] http://www.healthline.com/health/skin-disorders#8

❖ Skin malfunction

Acne, Cellulites, corns, calluses, hive, Ichthyosis, Melasma, stretch marks, varicose vein, wrinkles.

➜ Remedies: Skin detox, HSW, aloe vera gel, massage, and nutrition

❖ Bacteria, Virus, Parasites

Athlete's foot, chicken pox, dermatitis, eczema, impetigo, Lyme disease, moles, psoriasis, rashes, ringworm, scabies, seborrheic dermatitis, shingles, and warts.

➜ Remedies: Silver shield gel, herbal spray, golden salve, detoxification of the bowels, kidneys, and liver.

❖ Infection, Inflammation

Cancer, dermatitis, lupus, melanoma, moles, razor bumps, shingles, skin tags, and sunburn.

➜ Remedies: Silver shield gel, black sap, silver shield liquid (to drink), tea tree oil, and chlorophyll. Pho (Vietnamese soup) is one of the foods that could prevent these infections as it is cooked with beef bones, with plenty of bone marrow. Marrow produces red blood cells and some white blood cells, helping the immune system

Use good barrier creams to protect the skin from harmful sun rays.

Clear and release anger and resentments through forgiveness and love.

❖ Products banned by FDA in cosmetics[75]

The EU banned over 1000 chemicals in consumer products, while the FDA banned 9 of them. Read the labels to identify them.

1. Bithionol. It used to eliminate the smell in toilet products.
2. Chlorofluorocarbon propellants. Used in cosmetic aerosol. (21 CFR 700.23).
3. Chloroform. This causes cancer in animals.
4. Halogenated salicylanilides (di-, tri-, metabromsalan and tetrachlorosalicylanilide). Can cause skin disorder (21 CFR 700.15).
5. Hexachlorophene. Has a toxic effect to human skin and could damage mucous membranes. (21 CFR 250.250).
6. Mercury compounds. Used in eye products. It is toxic for the skin and brain. Mercury fillings in your teeth could be hazardous to your health. You need to clean them out.
7. Methylene chloride. Causes cancer in animals
8. Prohibited cattle materials: Mad cow disease.
9. Sunscreens in cosmetics. Sunscreen or sun protection is under different categories and isn't put in the cosmetics category.
10. Vinyl chloride. Causes cancer.
11. Zirconium-containing complexes. Toxic effect in animals' lungs and causes cancer.

---

[75]

http://www.fda.gov/Cosmetics/GuidanceRegulation/LawsRegulations/ucm127406.htm

What Does Your Body Really Need?
IN.FORM Chart

WHAT YOU'RE CRAVING	WHAT YOU NEED	FOODS CONTAINING NUTRIENTS
Chocolate	Magnesium	Raw nuts and seeds, legumes, fruit
Sweets	Chromium	Broccoli, grapes, cheese, dried beans, chicken
	Phosphorus	Chicken, beef, liver, poultry, fish, eggs, dairy, nuts, legumes
	Sulfur	Cranberries, horseradish, cruciferous, vegetables, kale, cabbage
	Tryptophan	Cheese, liver, lamb, spinach
Bread, toast	Nitrogen	High-protein foods: fish, meats, nuts, beans
Oily snacks, fatty foods	Calcium	Mustard and turnip greens, broccoli, kale, legumes, cheese, seasame seeds
Ice	Iron	Meat, fish, poultry, seaweed, greens, black cherries
Soda/Carbonated drinks	Calcium	Mustard and turnip greens, broccoli, kale, legumes, cheese, seasame seeds
Salty foods	Chloride	Raw goat milk, fish, unrefined sea salt
Pre-menstrual cravings	Zinc	Red meats, seafood, leafy vegerables, root vegetables
General Overeating	Silicon	Nuts, seeds: avoid refined starches
	Typtophan	Cheese, liver, lamb, spinach
	Tryosine	Vitamin C supplement: orange, green and red fruits and vegetables
Lack of Appetite	Vitamin Bl	Nuts, seeds, beans, liver
	Vitamin B3	Tuna, halibut, beef, chicken, turkey, pork, seeds, legumes
	Manganese	Walnuts, almonds, pecans, pineapple, blueberries
	Chloride	Raw goat milk, fish, unrefined sea salt

Chapter 11: Common Sense —Summary

1. Doc D.: Body ACE: Assimilate, Circulate and Eliminate. It does not matter what you eat, if your body can't process it. It could be harmful to you. When these three elements work in harmony, there should not be any problems and you will have good physical health.
2. Detoxification of the intestine and liver and metal detox from mercury fillings are important to know about to improve health.
3. Vitamins, minerals and trace minerals can't be produced by your body. They have to come from outside sources.
4. Your skin, your body is a sacred organization; it is the only one you have, at least in this reality. Treat them with love and respect and they will reward you with many years of happiness.
5. There are 44 types of skin disorders. Learn a few different tools to communicate with your body, such as muscle testing instead of just guessing, to prevent them.
6. Your skin (your body) daily needs: protein (for muscles: amino acids), fat (for protection, for fluid transportation of nutrients), carbohydrates (turn to glucose for energy), vitamins, minerals and trace minerals. Love, care and fun.

Chapter 12—Use All the Tools—Selectively!

Do what is best for you! The main point is to take good care of your body, mind and spirit.

> ➤ Modern technologies are excellent to detect irregular things in your physical body. Do checkups regularly. Your medical doctors are there to help you.
> ➤ Choose your foods and water and bless them before consuming to increase their nutrient benefits.
> ➤ Learn muscle testing or find good herbal company and herbalist to help you. Take vitamins and supplements daily to continue to maintain your body.
> ➤ There are many great tools and systems out there. Educate yourself to explore the benefits they can bring to you.

Everything around and inside us is energy and vibrates with certain frequencies. We believe learning energy for healing is essential for optimal living and well-being.

Our purpose of this book is to introduce you to some of the unique tools, processes, and programs you can use to improve your health and happiness.

Maybe there is nothing new in the universe, but we are convinced that the combination of many for Healing H.A.P.P.Y Bubbles systems is uniquely done by the company.

Some of the energy tools are:

Sound Healings

Sounds are vibrations. They have a very profound effect on the body, mind and spirit of humans. They have been used in societies for thousands of years in many forms and elements: [76]

- ➤ Buddhist Chanting.[77]
- ➤ Hindus Mantras Sanskrit.[78]
- ➤ Shamans Icaros (Melodies healing).[79]

➤ Solfeggio Frequencies

Ancient Solfeggio Frequencies

Solfeggio Scales can be traced back to a long time ago in the hymn of John the Baptist. It is used in sacred music to be in tune with the vibrations of the loving universe.

There are nine tunes including the six original ones

1- 174 HZ: Physical sense of security, safety. Could reduce pain energetically.

2- 285 HZ: Energy generating to rejuvenate and restructure

3- 396 HZ: Releasing emotional of guilt and fears, open path self-realization

4- 417 HZ: Clearing burdens of the past, connecting to new energy for mystic change

5- 528 HZ: Produce miracles in intention for Highest Good. Transform DNA

6- 639 HZ: Healing relationships with oneself and others

7- 741 HZ: Connect with power of SELF in image and expression

8- 852 HZ: Clarity in illusions and Holistic Realness to connect with the Source

9- 963 HZ: Joy of Coming Home

---

[76] http://www.soundhealersassociation.org/jonathan-goldman-9-elements-of-sound-healing

[77] https://en.wikipedia.org/wiki/Chant

[78] https://en.wikipedia.org/wiki/Mantra

[79] https://en.wikipedia.org/wiki/Icaro

Cleaning and Balancing the Chakras

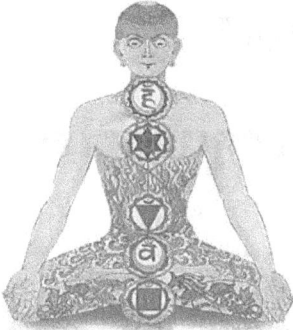

Self-Healing Secrets:
The Art of Cloning God!

Live a long time (100 years+) with Chakras balancing

Humans can live a long time in good health and strength if they know how to utilize the universal sources for Oneness.

Chakras are energy centers

❖ They are like the 7 senses. Without the 7 senses, there is no vision, no taste, no sound.

❖ Without the chakras, it there is no energy. It is blind, with no conscience, no feelings, and brain-dead.

❖ They are doorways of feelings in and out.

❖ There are 12 chakras: 7 inside the body, invisible, and 5 outside the body

❖ Each chakra has 49 levels of energy, altogether about 196 systems.

➤ Clearing Traumas

Traumas are feelings and emotions trapped in your brain at the subconscious level. Traumas are damaging because they reflect in your present behaviors and actions, and could hammer your efforts to have health and happiness.

Trauma can come in many forms:

- Pictures or sounds: repeating, recurrent pictures and sounds couple with shames, fears, hurts, pains and sufferings.
- Unresolved conflicts and anger: feeling frustrated, regrets, remorse triggered by smell or taste.
- Unsafe events or unstable environment generating fears and uncertainty.
- Hopeless, helpless, despair in anxiety, stressful situations.
- Serious illnesses or accidents affected the physical being.

People react differently in each situation; there is no right or wrong in keeping the trauma. It is personal impact depends on the individual psyche make-up, social and family influences, especially in childhood.

Brent Phillips, Awakening Dynamics, defines 3 levels of traumas: Emotional impact, Physical impact of trauma, and Cellular impact from the trauma.

Using Theta Healing and binaural beats in his Trauma Clearing program, Brent has helped hundreds of people, including me, to clear these dysfunctional blockages to be able to go forward with clarity and confidence. [80]

---

[80]   http://ywrdownloads.s3.amazonaws.com/Brent%20Phillips/overview-trauma-clearing.pdf

Heaven on Earth: Healing H.A.P.P.Y. Bubbles Systems™

Healing H.A.P.P.Y. Bubbles Systems stands for

H: Honorable;
A: Awesome;
P: Phenomenal;
P: Powerful and;
Y: You.

Earth and the Divine teams love and respect the human race as we are a dignified and honorable species.

Each of us carries a speck of the Divine inside and has the deepest desire to be all in Oneness.

Yet, Humans create duality and want to experience darkness and light in the physical form that makes each of us fascinatingly unique.

Healing H.A.P.P.Y Principles (ONE).

Happiness with Dignity.
Happiness has no meaning if its intention is to hurt or to be better than others. Your soul, your body, knows this. It is one of the four pillars of a person's life.

Dignity *means being worthy, having self-esteem, decency, morality, and trustworthiness.*

Happiness with Dignity
gives you the freedom to live your life the way you design it. It satisfies the "Divine Spark" inside you, and you can live life to the fullest of your values. You can give your contributions to the world in the most magnificent way.

Healing H.A.P.P.Y. Bubbles Principles (TWO.)

Love with Respect
Without respect, love is blurry and can be confused with physical desires and negative emotional attachments. Respect means you value others and are kind, truthful, and honest.

Without Love with Respect, you can't take good care of yourself, and therefore you can't take good care of others.

With Love and Respect, everything flourishes in the timeless, eternal values.

The connection to Earth and Divinity is always there and ready to be used. Many remember it; many forget it.

In 2012, a new dimension of awakening and awareness opened. We started remembering more and more and connecting with the Source more and more.

Where Does the Healing H.A.P.P.Y. Bubbles Systems ™ Come from?

When Vicki Tuong Vi went through her transformation from victimhood vibrations to vessel vibrations, she needed a safe, spiritual, heavenly place to rest, to heal, to learn, and to grow. Lazaris and her Higher Self provided her a portable, readily available sacred space to protect her.

Healing H.A.P.P.Y. Bubbles Principles (Three).

Beauty with Integrity

You are beautiful. Stop measuring your beauty by how your body and face compare to your "limited definition."

Beauty is the expression of the understanding of what life is and the uniqueness of your human experience.

***Beauty with Integrity** is the expression of wellness without judgment and competition. When you know this, your physical body will change to reflect yo inner beauty.*

Lazaris is a friend of human; he channeled through Jack Pursel since 1974. He is my spiritual teacher. [81]

Vicki then realized that she could program the healing codes in a system for faster results and asked for help. Her request is gifted.

It started with some of the Theta Healing Codes of Brent Phillips. And then blending with Earth energy.

Since then, Earth and Divine Teams have added many codes and are continuing to expand the systems.

---

[81] http://lazaris.com/

Healing H.A.P.P.Y. Bubbles Principles (FOUR).

Success with Honor

Creating **Success with Honor** is much easier and more fun than without it. It does not mean you give up your privacy. Honor means knowing and respecting your own privacy and the privacy of others and clearly defining the boundaries of trust, truth, and goodness.

It is a celebration of the mind. Your brain also knows this, and it gives you unlimited power to the creation and expansion of your imagination with continual growth.

Healing H.A.P.P.Y. Bubbles Systems Created by Earth and Divine Sources to help Human.

The systems are a huge set of prayers without borders. It is a synergy of Earth, Divinity, Human power, and Third power (extracted gems from experiences), healing sounds, Solfeggio and binaural beats, herbs, and vibrations. The system has many systems encoded within it and continues to change, grow, heal, balance, harmonize and expand.

The Systems Created not by Human, but for Human.

The Divine Teams include the following: the Creator, the Divine Source, God, Goddess All That Is, Earth's love and magical healing power, millions of Angels and Archangels, Guardian Angels, Spiritual Counselors, Guides, Unseen Friends, and many more known and unknown to humanity.

Healing H.A.P.P.Y. Bubbles Principles (FIVE & SIX).

Power with Responsibilities.

Without responsibilities, power has no values. It has no meaning, just a mighty destructive force, aimless; easily being manipulated.

Power is lasting when it is for the Highest Good of All.

Understanding with Uncertainty.

The only certain thing is uncertainty.

The abilities to handle uncertainty is the best certainty that one could have.

Humanity's life is dignified and honorable. Human has the power to choose to be in partnership with Earth and Divinity or not.

Without their permission, Divine's teams will not interfere.

After the bonds between the individual, Earth, and Divine's team are established. The relationships become inter-personal and intimate, including Higher Self, Soul, Future Self, Ego, Child, Adolescent, Magical Child and more.

Healing H.A.P.P.Y. Bubbles Principles (SEVEN).

Heaven on Earth in Human Form.

You can have it all. Wealth, Health, Beauty, Happiness, Dignity, Honor in all 7 aspects of Life: Health, Career, Finance, Society, Spirit, Family & Friends, Love (Added by Mr. G.)

Access to the Healing H.A.P.P.Y. Bubbles Systems. ™ by joining at:

www.FunHappyStore.com

The Divine teams' choice is to love human beings and to help them evolve to higher levels of awareness, awakening to become Oneness.

Human understanding is different from Divine Intelligence.

When humans align their purposes and principles with the Divine, everything changes; life becomes "eternal" with goodness, truth, beauty, and fun with ease and grace.

Beautiful Truths of the Universe [82]

We are here to learn to take *good* care of ourselves.
If you do not know how to take care of yourself or don't take good care of yourself, who is going to do it for you?

We are here to learn to have fun.

Taking good care of yourself is fun and exciting. Knowing yourself, learning other aspects affecting your being is fascinating and ever changing. Knowing how to have fun allows you to create and expand your ability without limits.

You are not alone.

You are never alone; you only mistakenly think that you are. There is so much help, all the time, 24/7, anywhere you go. Simply allow and ask for help. Help will come always; it never fails. You are a Speck of Divinity of the Creator of the Divine Teams. Open your heart to allow, receive, and accept help. In turn, learn to be a team player and help others in need.
You are loved for no *reason*.

The Divine Teams choose to love you; they love you for no reason. You can't lose or forget this love. It is always there. Simply remember it, and in turn, help others to remember this love, too.

You matter. You are valued, and you are valuable.

You add value to your world. You matter. You might make mistakes, but it doesn't mean you don't have values.

---

[82] www.Lazaris.com

Inside the Healing H.A.P.P.Y. Bubbles Systems™

Learn Energy Healing for Health, Beauty and Wellness.

Your body is a sacred temple. Nothing can affect it unless you allow.

This includes Divine Teams. They can't help you if you don't allow them to. They can help you to rid of Illnesses, negative emotions, mature your negative ego, creating miracles, wealth and happiness.

Future books:

Say Yes 2 Happiness for Awesome Lifetime Success.

A Penny for Happiness – Children's book.

The systems have millions of complex codes including the following important words and concepts and protocols:

- Awake, aware, safety, security, protection, prevention, Heaven failsafe
- Clean, clear, heal.
- Release, forgive and forget, lift up the shames, healing the hurts, clearing the pains, cleaning the sufferings.
- Allow, activate, download, infuse, circulate.
- Install new beliefs that are permanent, complete, continuous, automatic, and on auto-pilot.
- Celebrate, envision, joy, gratitude. Flow out Healing H.A.P.P.Y. Bubbles to the world.

❖ How Do I Use It?

The system is very easy to use; even a kid can do it.

- Connect to Heaven and Earth.
- Activate Healing H.A.P.P.Y. Bubbles Systems.
- Connect Bubbles to you and ask for desired help.

There are many applications; here are a few things you can use H.A.P.P.Y. Bubbles for:

- Cleaning and clearing the environment, and your body of radiations, viruses, harmful chemicals, harmful bacteria, parasites, mold, etc.
- Clearing adverse weather to calm weather.
- Changing the water structure to be safe to drink.
- Repairing your car; filling the gas tank in an emergency.
- Calling for help in and to avoid adverse situations.
- Sending out 10,000 blessings (Sylvia Oga Ortiz).
- Asking the Divine to flow millions of H.A.P.P.Y. Bubbles to people or countries where and when as needed.
- Healing illnesses of your physical body or loved ones.
- Manifest money flowing into your bank accounts.
- Protect your luggage against lost or damages.
- Protect your children, loved ones.
- Create miracles.

- And much, much more.

❖ A Few Wonders

It was said that human being is a self-generated thought in a place between time and space. The amazing thing about this species is the complexity and sophistication in the simplest way.

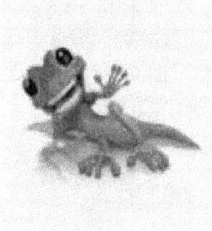

> There are so many visible things and so many invisible things, from the physical wonders to the aura field, to the ethereal body, to the psychic body, to the emotional body, to the mental body, to the spiritual body, and to energy fields.

> There are many things you can do to enhance skin health: herbal medicines, modern techniques, sound healings, muscle testing, psychic reading, lucid dreaming, binaural beats, Solfeggio frequencies, chanting, religions, meditations, society, relationship, music, EFT (Emotional Freedom Technique), and many more.

> There are hundreds of energy vortexes in the Chakras system. Energy flow through over 75,000 *Nadis channels* to every cell. Learning to balance and harmonize these energies is beneficial for your health.

> The wonders are infinite. YOU are infinite! Enjoy!

Chapter 12: Use All these Tools, Selectively! —Summary Box

1. Taking good care of yourself is knowing yourself: what you want, need and what is good for you. It means being well aware of the Is, techniques, and programs available to be the best you can be.

2. Know that there are many excellent systems out there. Choose and combine a few suitable processes and make them your daily routine.

3. All of which is responding to the need to connecting with the Universe and connecting with each other. All is about to live your Life to the fullest and to enjoy the journey of Coming Home to Oneness.

4. The principles of them are the same, but the journey is an individual undertaking. The creation, your creation, is endless.

5. This book serves as the first book in the series to share and to work with you in love and beauty for your face and skin. We hope you enjoy it and use all the tools you need to be where you want to be!

Inspiration Quotes

Thank you to many people who love me, believe in me amd support me; despite all of my shortcomings!
This is just a short list of their beautiful thoughts to share with the readers and the world.

> *It does not matter how much money you are making; it does matter what kind of person you are becoming.* **"Dr. 3Es"**

> *I just want to be Happy!!!* **"Matt E."**

> *I am a happy, easy going person!* **"Theresa H."**

> *There was an accident yesterday involved a police officer. We just want to make sure you are safe* **"A Police Officer"**
> *"A symbol Healing H.A.P.P.Y. Bubbles™" dedicating for safety, security, prevention, protection & Heaven fail safe was created to honor the officer. www.HealingHAPPYBubbles.com."*

> *God is the vast equitable of equitability (Công Bình and Bình đẳng)* **"Mr. Hoang Chuong"**

Everyone has a book inside them **"Steve Harrison, Quantum Leap"**

You never know whose Life you touch until you share. Go ahead go sharing! **"Doc D. Super Group NJ"**

H.A.P.P.Y. Bubbles Kids Adventures **"Jenny JJ – 8-year-old"**

Writing a book changed my life **"Jack Canfield-Chicken Soup for the Soul"**

Have you ever feel sad, unhappy? What do you do then? **"MRE – 7-year-old"**
"Yes, I feel sad and unhappy sometimes. When it happens, I acknowledge the feelings, then I release them by sending out to the Universe to transform them to beautiful energies with 10,000 times of blessings. Then I download, install Magic Circles (HHB) and 9-9-6-1, thank you God; for Love and Happiness. And I go and continue to have fun!" **"HHB-VTV"**
"You don't have to be unhappy to be happy. Remember the Love to forgive, forget, release, refresh. Everything is OK, everything is always OK" **"Angels Vibrations HHB"**

We love computers. Technologies are a big part of Human Future. *"Gary & Kathy AVTECHUSA.com"*

I retired my sufferings forever! I matured my negative ego to a supportive, mature, loving with a sense of humor, wise, beautiful, healthy & happy awesome EGO! Yeah! *"Earth Love - HHB"*

One of my favorite quotes comes from a Tom Hanks' movie, Forrest Gump: "Life is like a box of chocolates, you never know what you are going to get". To me this says, it's about the experience, the journey, the choice. It reminds us all that it's all about choice and the choice you make doesn't really matter but that there is a choice and that the best part is all inside. Go discover your sweetness. ordinary blessings, *"Cheryl from AZ"*

Money is Oneness, when it is for doing good. The more money you make; the more people you can help. *"Vicki Tuong Vi"*

"Welcome Change because Change is really the only constant that you can count on!" *"Angela T"*

"I am grateful for my coaching opportunities. I welcome the heavenly ideas that pop into my head!" *"Tamra -www.myspeakersheet.com"*

We are here to help. Call me anytime! *"Scott T. Nature's Sunshine Regional Manager"*

Buying a home is more than having a place to live. It is to expand your horizon of creativity and happiness *"Chris Goodson, Goodson Law Firm, NJ"*

Go JV partners. You don't have to do it alone! *"Milana & Rich"*

"Welcome Change because Change is really the only constant that you can count on!" "Angela T"

"Life is beautiful, so go ahead, empty your cup and go Live Life beautifully, today and every day!" *"Angels Vibrations HHB-VTV"*

Divine Intelligence and Human Understanding are two different things **"Brent Phillips"**

Go into the quantum field and let the energy carry you **"Dr. Karl Wolfe – www.karlwolfe.com"**

"If Opportunity Came Disguised as Temptation, Then It Would Only Need to Knock Once!" **"Angela T"**

We want to ensure your success. Take the imperfect actions **"Barry, Roger, Mike, Tammy"**

I surround me in beauty. I go to sleep in beauty and wake up in beauty. **"Dr. Karl Wolfe – www.karlwolfe.com"**

I found this penny on the ground yesterday, I am giving it to you, I think it will make you very happy! **"Se – 5-year-old"**
"Yes, indeed, it made me very happy, I save it and call it: "A Penny for Happiness" It is my next children book. Thank you. ☺"

225

Endnote: Why Did We Write this Book?

Hello, this is Vicki (Tường Vi) Eaton. Thank you very much for your interest in Healing H.A.P.P.Y. Bubbles Systems™— Eternal Youth Secrets: How to Have Beautiful Hair, Glowing Skin at Any Age.

In Asia, Good Fortune, Prosperity, and Longevity are our cultural traditions, which are great, of course, but times have changed! We want to live long lives and be wealthy, happy, and beautiful, too. When we look at Shou Ông Thọ (the Longevity God of the three Gods: Blessings, Prosperity, and Longevity) with the big forehead, we say, "Hmmm, how can we look better today in modern times?" (Google Fu Lu Shou and you can see his picture online). Shou's picture is on the left, below, and Fu Lu Shou's picture is next to it on the right, below.

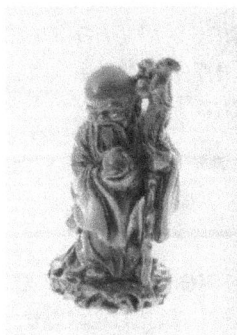

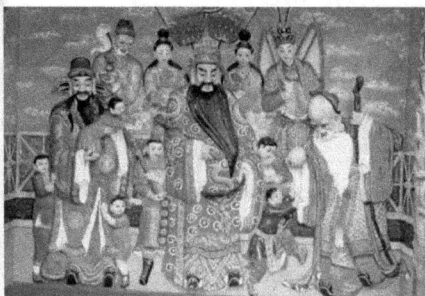

For all we know, most everyone, we think, wants to look beautiful no matter how old they are. My mother was in her 90s, in poor health, and quite fragile, an invalid suffering and in physical pain 24/7. She passed away in 2013 after several praying sessions connecting with the Divine, which was arranged for me by my friend Sylvia Ortiz.

The connection with Divinity allowed her to link back with her Higher Self to understand death. This helped her remember her human dignity and honor. She left her ailing physical body in peace with awareness, no pains, no sufferings afterward.

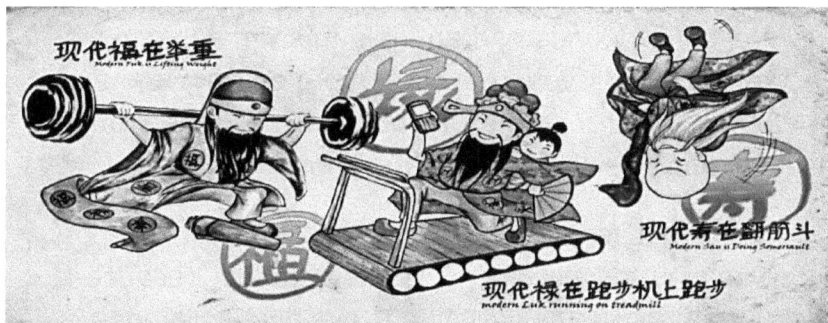

Seeing our mother's departing transformation, we said to each other, "We want to be able to be strong in our old age. We want to swim, run the treadmill, do jumping jacks, and look beautiful until the day we leave Earth. We don't want to wait to die by getting old and be a burden to our loved ones. When it is time for us to leave the physical body, we want to just 'Poof' and go, leaving this physical body in minutes. No fuss, no pains, no nursing home!"

So, my coauthors and I developed a system to maintain good health and a method to maintain a beautiful face, skin, and hair. We put these techniques to the test with the intention of publishing a series of books and DVDs about longevity, beauty, success, and good health in the near future.

We hired people to draw a modern version of Fu Lu Shou, showing him lifting weights, running on the treadmill, and doing a somersault. Hilarious! The picture shows the fun... so much fun!!!

227

After my car accident a decade ago, I was overweight and ridden with many illnesses: high blood pressure, borderline diabetes, acid reflux, asthma…you name it. I did not want to take medicine, so I begged my wonderful Doctor Krupp[83] to give me a few months to find alternative solutions. He agreed. I turned to Vietnamese medicine, Eastern techniques, natural medicine, and holistic healing.

So far, I've lost 40+ pounds and am able to swim nonstop for an hour or more. I look younger, have more energy, and am feeling healthier. I jump on the trampoline almost every day, use massage, and stretch daily (see the photo below, left).

I even enrolled in Lifeguard Certification class, but did not pass the swimming rescue test. It is okay, though because I continue to use the systems daily to achieve my health goals.

I am currently taking herbal vitamins, minerals, and trace minerals from a few select companies and using muscle

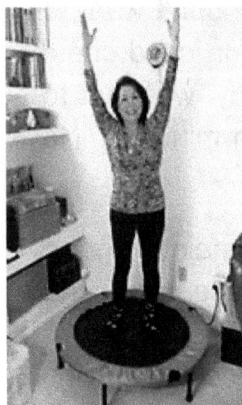

67 year old lady
on the trampoline
after traumas clearing

testing to confirm the supplements my body needs. It is working. The only medicine I am taking now is for high blood pressure. In 2015, I cleared my traumas with the Theta Healing of Brent Phillips. It changed my life completely to a higher dimension. I was able to connect with the Source and co-create the H.A.P.P.Y. Bubbles systems!

My coauthors and I wrote this book and made the DVD to share with you the fun, techniques, programs, and processes we are using.

---

[83]   http://local.yahoo.com/info-18183609-krupp-edward-do-crescent-internal-medicine-grp-montclair

In addition, we would love to present the connections we have with the Divine, Mother Earth, plants and the animal kingdom in the Healing H.A.P.P.Y. Systems ™ to you. It is up to you to apply the methods to create your own reality the way you wanted.

Face massaging, exercising, and acupressure are not new, yet they are proven, effective techniques. We did not invent them; instead, we combined and modified them according to our needs. We are not beauty experts, medical professionals, or writers; we are just ordinary people like you. If we can use the system to improve our health and have beautiful faces and skin with good health and happiness, you can, too.

When Ngọc Ánh (one of the coauthors) fell and became paralyzed, she used a combination of modern technologies, natural herbs, traditional medicine, and Energy Healing to help herself. Today, her hair has grown back, the numbness in her hands is gone, she can drive her velosolex, ☺ and she is normal and healthy again.

Minh Trang, another coauthor, is in her 20s but wants to participate. She majors in English and business and will be the translator for the book and DVD into Vietnamese.

We hope you find the information helpful. We use organic, essential oil mixtures. You can use these formulas with your current products or create your own mixtures. Available resources are everywhere, online or offline. They might help you. Like anything else in life, apply common sense and always do the best for your body and skin health.

Customer Service

Thank you for allowing us the opportunity to share these techniques with you.

It is a natural desire to want to be healthy, live long, prosper, and be beautiful for as long as we can. The tools of having beautiful skin to match your inner beauty are now in your hands.

We hope you'll enjoy them as much as we do.

We are not beauty experts, medical professionals, or writers; we are just a happy bunch of people who love life, value relationships, and believe in doing good things. We want to live hundreds of years in a 30-year-old body with a beautiful face and good health, and be rich, too.

Crazy? Unrealistic? Not Doable? Well, we don't know. We just know we are having so much fun doing this and learning something new by connecting and sharing with you.

We hope you feel the same.

You have nothing to lose with our 30-Day Product Return/Exchange Policy. If you do not like the products; simply send them back with proof of purchase to:

Customer Service, The Eternal Youth Methods
4 Beaverbrook Road
Lincoln Park, NJ 07035

We will send your refund to you minus shipping, handling and restocking charges. If you receive a damaged or defective item, we will be happy to exchange it for you immediately.

Healing H.A.P.P.Y. Bubbles Systems ™
Personal Development & Enhancement to Live
Life in Beauty, Truth and Goodness

"Not a perfect system, but a Complete system!"

To promote Awareness, Awakening of Conscious
Choices to the World for the Highest Good of All.

Healing H.A.P.P.Y. Bubbles principles:
Happiness with Dignity, Love with Respect
Success with Honor, Beauty with Integrity,
Power with Responsibility, Understanding with Uncertainty.

Three levels of programs:

Level 1: The Eternal Youth Methods ™ – Learn the secrets of Happiness with Dignity to be stronger and healthier every day. Master muscle testing to tap into the Healing H.A.P.P.Y Bubbles System ™ - Victor level in Hawkins scale.

Level 2: Dance with Beauty & Grace Speaker Program **Healers & Practitioners – Vessel level in Hawkins scale.**

Level 3: Healing H.A.P.P.Y. Bubbles Presenter – The system is a synergy of unlimited and mystical energies, created to help human to connect with the Source on their journey to come Home. As such, the program teaches human to be co-creators and Presenter of **Angels Earth & Divinity Vibrations in Human Form – Heaven on Earth.**

For more information, please visit
FunHAPPYstore.com

Making Conscious Choices of Good Health & Happiness is up to you.

Human beings have the ability to choose.
This is what makes us human. Plants and animals do not have te ability to choose.

Human beings have the freedom to choose.
You have the freedom to choose whether you know it or not. If you don't choose, something, someone will choose for you, and you may not like it.

Allow, accept, & receive spiritual help.
Allowing help from the Divinity and Earth–who love you—is different than asking only for help. When you allow help and are willing to accept and receive help, there are things that happen to benefit you whether you consciously know it or not.

Introducing the Coauthors

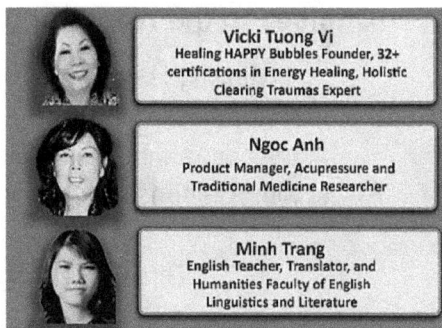

| Vicki Tuong Vi |
| Healing HAPPY Bubbles Founder, 32+ certifications in Energy Healing, Holistic Clearing Traumas Expert |

| Ngoc Anh |
| Product Manager, Acupressure and Traditional Medicine Researcher |

| Minh Trang |
| English Teacher, Translator, and Humanities Faculty of English Linguistics and Literature |

Healing H.A.P.P.Y. Bubbles Systems™ Eternal Youth Secrets: How to Have Beautiful Hair, Glowing Skin at Any Age.

Divine Teams
Creator, Divine, Source, God, Goddess All That Is.
Millions of Angels and Archangels
Unseen Friends, Spiritual Counselors, Higher Self, Healing Guides
and many more known or unknown divinities.

Future Publications

1.   Say Yes to Happiness with Dignity for Awesome Lifetime Success.

- ❖ Self-Healing Longevity
- ❖ Relationships
- ❖ Total Health
- ❖ Society
- ❖ Published date: Nov 2016

2.   Learning Energies Healing to Clear Your Traumas Permanently.

- ❖ Clear traumas, shocks, and cellular traumas permanently
- ❖ Release hurts, pain and suffering
- ❖ Reprogram your subconscious with Vessel energies for Success with Honor
- ❖ Download and install the *Divine Dictionary* and sync to yours

3. Divine Learning Skills using healing sounds, Solfeggio, binaural beats, brain optimization, and more!

Can we reverse the aging process? Yes, we can try! With Fun & Elegance & Excellence!!!

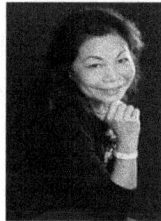

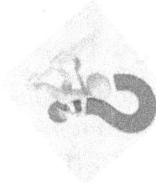

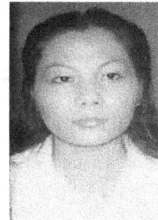

Acknowledgments

There are too many to list...this is just a short list.
If we missed anyone, please forgive us!

- ❖ Dr. D and Family – "Super Group of NJ": Candace, Barbara M., Barbara, Batoul, Linda
- ❖ Nature's Sunshine Company and Scott Terry and Coaches
- ❖ Gary Mao and Kathy Fan: AVTechUSA.com
- ❖ Chris Goodson, Esq. Angela and Teams
- ❖ Theresa Nga and Family and Ted Thanh Mai
- ❖ Editors: Expert Publishing VW, Madalyn Stone- Angela Thomas
- ❖ Sam and MS Jewelry
- ❖ Linda and friends and "H.A.P.P.Y. Bubbles kids.
- ❖ Mike, Barry, Roger, Tammy Group and Members
- ❖ Dr. Karl Wolf – Karlwolf.com – Movement Feedback Holography
- ❖ Steve Harrison, Jack Canfield – Quantum Leap and Coaches
- ❖ Lazaris – Spiritual Human Friend
- ❖ Brent Phillips – Awakening Dynamics – The Formula for Miracles
- ❖ Dr. Paul Scheele – Learning Strategies
- ❖ Daniel the Healer – Danielthehealer.com
- ❖ JV Rich and Milana and JV groups
- ❖ Cha và 2 mẹ tôi : Văn Láng Thị Na Thị Chắt
- ❖ MM. Văn Đông, Văn Tiến, Thanh Tuyền
- ❖ Mlles. Thị Tới, Thị Tấn, Kim Thoa
- ❖ Mme Kim Lan, M. Lân Trương and Mlle. Luân Vũ
- ❖ Mlle. Phương, MM. Bùi Nghĩa, Phan Toại
- ❖ Dr. Ed and Lorena, Madeline, Sebastian, Oliver, Maxwell
- ❖ M. Matthew and Janine, Mason
- ❖ Mlles Ngọc Phượng, Tuyết Nhung, Thanh Tuyền
- ❖ Mlles Thùy Anh, Minh Ngọc,
- ❖ MM. Đình Duy, Bùi Nam, Đạt Long
- ❖ MM. Duy Minh, Eric Phùng

- Nghĩa, Quân Hướng Việt Restaurant
- MM. Trần Giáo, Nguyễn Giáo, Thịnh
- Hà and Family
- Nghĩa, Quân Hướng Việt Restaurant
- MM. Trần Giáo, Nguyễn Giáo, Thịnh
- Harvey Vedder, Judy Vedder: IridologyNYC.com
- Deirdre Anderson: HunterdonZumba.com
- Debra, Kathleen, Rebecca
- Lorraine Henrich, Marcella Hilferty, Martina Ruddock
- Sylvia Vega-Ortiz – Dick and Nancy Weber
- Jeffrey and GailAnne, Valerie Lemme
- Dr. Krupp – Montclair, NJ – Dr. Sluka – Bloomingdale, NJ
- Pamela, Frank, Kathy, Edgar and Staffs MVC
- Mary Jane and Ron – George and Gail – Bob Heilig (NAP)
- Rob Bell: GreenBirdieVideo.com and Network Lambertville and Vinny
- Kenton Johnson: ProsperSystems.biz
- Earth and Divinity Teams
- Personal friends and counsellors

Journaling Your Progress!

Name: _____ Date: _____

Your Picture

Before

Your Picture

After

Take your picture before and after.

Find a picture of yourself when you were younger; this is your goal, how you want your fresh face to look.

Buy a notebook.

Journal your progress each week.

Eat healthy; chew your food and drink your liquids.

Take care of yourself.

Bless yourself every day.

Release emotional stress by sending back 10,000 Blessings to the sender, including yourself.

Have fun in everything you do!

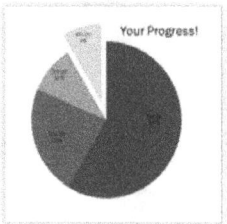

Above All: LIVE! APPLY WHAT YOU LEARN NOW!

Journaling & Notes

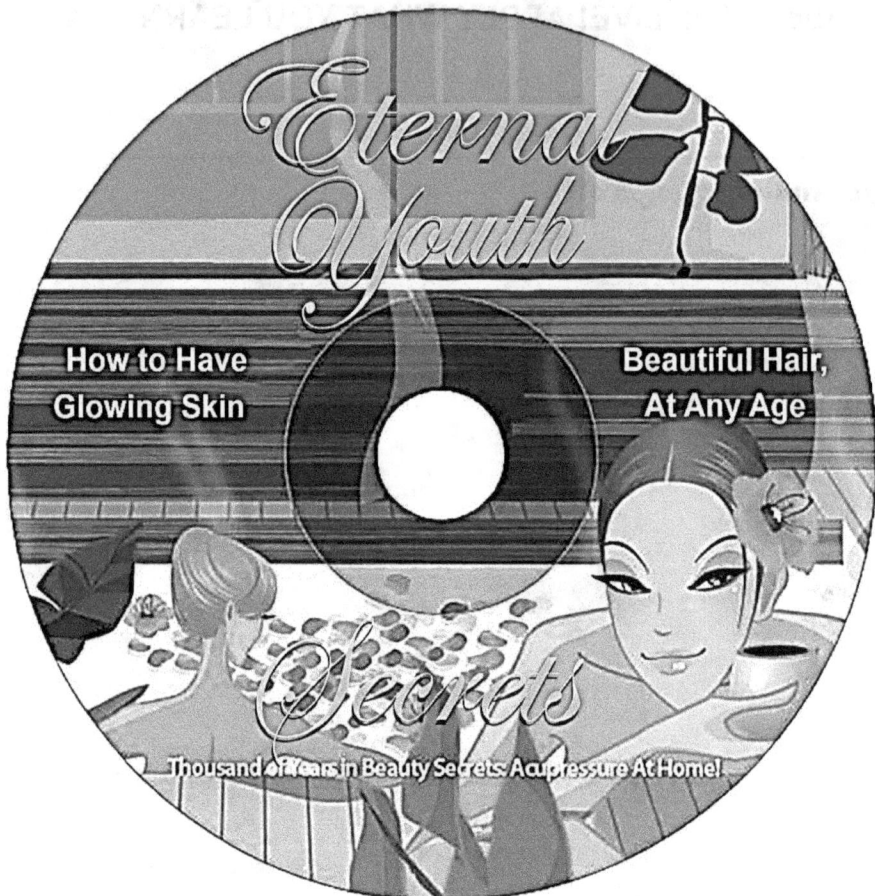

Eternal Youth

How to Have Glowing Skin

Beautiful Hair, At Any Age

Secrets

Thousand of Years in Beauty Secrets Acupressure At Home!

Order your Video at
www.FunHappyStore.com

For Nature's Sunshine products, sign up with Vicki Eaton
Nature's Sunshine In-Form Coach
ID # 2948007

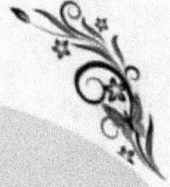

You are Beautiful,
Life is Beautiful,
So Go Ahead, Empty Your Cup;
And Go Live Life Beautifully
Today & Everyday!

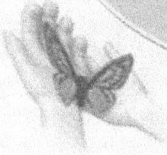

Human has the power to choose, where as animals and plants do not!

www.HealingHAPPYBubbles.com

Choose to be healthy, happy and successful. Choose to do good for our own Self, then for the world.
Choose → Decide → Take Actions
Then sit back, relax and watch all the magic happen!

www.ingramcontent.com/pod-product-compliance
Lightning Source LLC
Chambersburg PA
CBHW062215270326
41930CB00009B/1739